OPTIMAL BRE

The Way You Breathe Cc
Or Make You Well!

... HELP YOU SING BETTER • SPEED YOUR RECOVERY FROM STRESS
++ EXTEND YOUR LIFE ++
& THOUSANDS OF WONDERFUL LIFE ENHANCING BENEFITS.
Breath is life.

by

Michael Grant White
LMBT • NE • OBDMT

Did you know that Optimal Breathing does not come naturally.
It is as skill.
We ALL need to breathe and we ALL can learn to breathe
much better.

ISBN 1-883417-06-6

Author of:

Secrets of Optimal Breathing® Development
including Building Healthy Lungs, Naturally

OPTIMAL BREATHING®

The Way You Breathe Can Make You Sick.

Or Make You Well!

© 2004 by Michael Grant White, LMBT • NE • OBDMT
Edited by Jan Jenson & Kay Graybeal
Design & layout by Jan Jenson • Vizual Explorations
http://www.breathing.com/theway.htm - download a FREE pdf
version of this book (customizable for your bs.!)

Copyright & Disclaimer

Medical Disclaimer: Any exercise or advice given in this book is not intended to replace the services of your physician, or to provide an alternative to professional medical treatment. This book offers no diagnosis or treatment for any specific medical problem. Where we suggest the possible usefulness of certain practices in relation to certain illnesses or symptoms, it is for educational purposes — either to explore the relationship of natural breathing to health or to expose the reader to alternative healing approaches.

Anyone with a serious medical or psychological problem such as heart disease, high blood pressure, cancer, mental illness, or recent abdominal or chest surgery, should consult their physician before pursuing this information.

The Secrets of Developing Optimal Breathing manual focuses on developing mechanical breathing function. Building Healthy Lungs Naturally (available both inside and separate from the Secrets manual) will give you key nutritional information in expanded formats.

Always consult a health professional when any illness develops.
Second and third opinions are often quite valuable especially
when drugs and or surgery are involved.
Don't just "go with" what you're told first.
— Michael Grant White, Optimal Breathing®

Goals and purposes of Optimal Breathing®

• To give new hope to the sick and dying and internal power to those in need.

• To educate and attract people who want to take responsibility for their health and longevity.

• To help people to realize that all non-surgically altered and congenitally normal humans breathe the same way and that anyone can learn to breathe better..

• To bring awareness to simple approaches and practices everyone can experiment with to find what works best for them with their unique health, performance and life extension aspirations taken in account.

• To guide people into realizing through their personal experience and the experiences of dear friends and loved ones, that the way they breathe is so powerful and important, that it becomes a major priority to want to inspire others to know what they know about optimal breathing development.

• To show traditional and alternative health professionals and any of the helping/training professions exactly how to utilize the fundamentals of Optimal Breathing® so they can enhance their system(s) with ours and apply their new holistic paradigm for all patients, clients, teachers and students unique needs?

• To get people to realize that emergent patterns, rising out of our primitive and enduring "suck, swallow, breathe" reflexes greatly influence the who we are and what we do as we unfold our lives one breath at a time. With Optimal Breathing as our foundation, we have a lot more to say about our present and future than we ever thought possible.

• To restore or strengthen our faith in who we are and the Source from where we came.

Michael Grant White

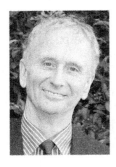

Michael is one of the most unusual teachers in the world today, with more than 30 years of research and development of breathing. Mike is one of those rare individuals whose destiny was revealed to him at a very young age - when he was asked to sing for his grammar school student body. Subsequent physical abuse left him unable to sing and what followed has been a quest to regain his singing voice and inner sense of wholeness. Learning what did not work was almost as beneficial as learning what did work.

Michael's students include a wide range of individuals, business executives, personal and spiritual growth seekers, amateur and professional athletes, speakers and singers and many types of holistic health practitioners.

Educator with Breathing Focus

Mike is an educator who uses breathing development for stress management, superior health, emotional balance, self expression and personal power. He combines key elements of Christianity, Hatha, Tibetan and Kundalini Yoga, Pranayama, Chi Kung, Massage and bodywork therapy, meditations, Chi Kung, Tai Chi, Karate, Reichian Therapy, Radiance Breathwork[a], Rebirthing[a], meditation, chanting, toning, operatic and public speaking training, and nutrition. He is a founding member of the Association Of Humanistic Psychology Somatics Community Steering committee, a former member of Unity Center, Walnut Creek, Ca and a member of The Health Medicine Forum of Lafayette, CA.

He delivers lectures and workshops worldwide and uses his Secrets of *Optimal Breathing® Development* manual and recorded breathing exercise cassettes to support his work. He has appeared on the Gary Null show, and national cable TV 's *Lifetime* Channel.

Articles written by Mike have appeared in **Massage** Magazine, *Women's Sports and Fitness, Boardroom Reports*, and a children's book created by the *Disney Channel.* He is quoted in a Rodale book for women titled **Natural Calm** (2001). **Optimal Breathing®** is listed in Rodale Press' book on alternative healing titled **Alternative Cures** (2000).

Current Research

Currently Michael is working with some of the nation's top physicians and behavior and alternative health specialists to expand the use of **Optimal Breathing©** in new and exciting areas of therapy, voice and music, sports performance and personal growth.

Optimal Breathing® helps eliminate the barriers that prevent vocalists and athletes from reaching peak performance and can help everyone achieve their maximum potential through astonishing healing techniques and exercises for many health conditions   How's YOUR breathing?   Take   our   online   tests   at   **http:// www.breathing.com/results.htm** then choose the health condition or performance goals that you wish to address.

To contact Michael Grant White at **Optimal Breathing®**:
http://www.breathing.com
Phone: 1-866-694-6425 (866-MyInhale)

Table of Contents

Results from over 40,000 free breathing tests at www.breathing.com/tests.htm have convinced me that poor breathing is connected with virtually every illness or compromised human ability.

Breath is life. Did you know that Optimal Breathing® does not come naturally? It is a skill. We ALL need to breathe and we ALL can learn to breathe much better.

• What's Really Killing Us??? Leading causes of death in the U.S.

• Improved breathing can dramatically influence your life skills in these waysÉ

• Rosetta Stone - the story of a key

• Definition of the "breathing reflex"

• Factors affecting or affected by breathing

• Detoxification & proper nutrition

• Breathing problems begin BEFORE pregnancy:

• Foods & drinks that are harmful to your health

• Mike's favorite breathing exercise – "The Squeeze & Breathe® Technique"

INTRODUCTION

OPTIMAL BREATHING®, The Way You Breathe Can Make You Sick. It Can Also Make You Well examines the obvious and subtle signals related to present and potential breathing problems and explains why making improvements in your breathing mechanics, diet, toxicity levels, attitude and environment can produce huge changes in your life.

First, learn why to improve your breathing. Then, if you have an interest, you can take our beginning and advanced training and become certified to teach others how to improve their breathing. Breathing is generic to all humanity, therefore all health care professionals will find breathing development a valuable addition to the services they offer.

You may want to invest in our most popular home study training program #176 DVD or video (http://www.breathing.com/video-manual-1-2.htm) and/or attend the Optimal Breathing® School (apprentice and advanced levels) Check our calendar of events for the days and place of the next scheduled Optimal Breathing School: http://www.breathing.com/school/main.htm

EVERYONE can greatly improve their breathing! But why bother learning about breathing at all?

I believe that barring harmful accidents, birth defects and certain surgeries, practically every health goal CAN be

8

attained with a holistic combination of breathing development, cleansing, fasting, organic live nutrition, vitamin/mineral supplements, prayer and meditation, positive daily affirmations, pure water, clean air and living environment, optimal ergonomics and moderate exercise.

My *Secrets of Developing Optimal Breathing®* manual fully explores the vast range of breathing development techniques developed from my 30 years experience, and utilizes more than 40,000 test results from my online breathing tests. This enables me and the **Optimal Breathing® School** staff and graduates to help others with singing, athletics, meditating, laughing, bliss, crying, speaking out, performing delicate tasks, recovering from stress of habitual activities that cause shallow or distorted breathing, the quickest and most thorough healing of wounds and illnesses, physical, emotional and spiritual.

Building Healthy Lungs, Naturally goes into greater detail and show you how to improve your breathing and quality of life even more by addressing nutrition, detoxification and relevant clinical studies...

"Breathing properly allows us to run the full range of emotions, and yet come back to deep peace, etc. We become able, like the animals in the wild, to shake off our stress, become calm and recover in the shortest possible times. "Reasonable" is defined by our individual values. Hopefully we seek those values that support our highest way of being. If this is not achieved then it is not optimal because states of

9

peace, love and joy are what my research has lead me to believe is the physical body's natural state of being and allows for the longest and most satisfying life."
— **Michael Grant White**

Use our comprehensive way of evaluating your breathing!
FREE BREATHING TESTS:
http://www.breathing.com/tests.htm

Chapter 1
ARE YOU AT RISK?

Did you know?

☆ Did you know that traditional medical, therapy and alternative health professionals are often taught incorrect ways of how breathing should look, feel and sound? This fosters a distorted perception of what is considered normal. More about this in my *Secrets of Optimal Breathing® Development* manual.

☆ Heart attacks, cancer, strokes, pneumonia, asthma, speech problems and almost every disease known to mankind are made worse or improved by your breathing and the quality of your respiration? Do you know the 30-year 5,200 person Framingham Study proved that how well your lungs function is a major factor of how long you live? This Study and follow-ups proved the association between impaired pulmonary function and all causes of death. *"This Study focused on the long-term predictive power of vital capacity (how deep is your inhale) and forced exhale volume (FEV-1) as the primary markers for life span. This pulmonary (lung) function measurement appears to be an indicator of general health and vigor and literally is a measure of living capacity."* - Dr. William B. Kannel.

☆ Did you know your body removes waste products by first combining those wastes with oxygen?

☆ The average person reaches peak respiratory function and lung capacity in their mid 20's. Then they begin to lose respiratory capacity between 10% and 27% for every decade of life! So, unless you are doing something to maintain or improve your breathing capacity, it will decline, and with it, your general health and your life expectancy. More about this in the *Secrets* manual.

☆ Do you know that almost every illness known to humanity has, at some point, been cured by proper breathing? When you look deeper into breathing issues, it's no surprise that in sufficient quantities, oxygen kills ALL germs, bacteria and viruses. This is not new information. Otto Warburg received the 1931 Nobel prize for proving that cancer can not flourish in a high oxygen environment. Plus, we now know that most heart attacks are caused by lack of oxygen.

"When you are out of breath nothing else matters" — a slogan of the American Lung Association.
☆ Did you know that as oxygen levels decline in polluted cities, reduced oxygen levels causes or worsens feelings of anxiety, desperation and heightened sense of your survival being threatened?

What's Really Killing Us?
The Center for Disease Control and the National Center for Health Statistics showed the fourth leading cause of death in this country in 1994 was emphysema and bronchitis. Elsewhere reported, asthma has increased 66% in the last ten years. When the oxygen supply decreases, the heart must work harder. Heart attacks stem largely from lack of oxygen. Also, germs, viruses, and bacteria are anaerobic: they cannot survive in high concentrations of oxygen.

We are bombarded daily with information on foods, exercise, alcohol consumption and smoking. We all know what we should do to improve our health.

But who talks about your breathing? Who teaches you HOW to do it properly?

We all breathe 4-20 times a minute, all day long. If we stop we die.

What can you learn about breathing that will improve your health?

☆ Do you know that in spite of so-called modern medicine, most categories of illness are getting worse and increasing in numbers and severity? That's largely because drugs and surgery treat the symptoms, not the causes of illness.

Leading Causes of Death in the U.S. in 2001

Heart Disease: 700,142

Cancer: 553,768

Stroke: 163,538

Chronic lower respiratory diseases: 123,013

Accidents (unintentional injuries): 101,537

Diabetes: 71,372

Influenza/Pneumonia: 62,034

Alzheimer's disease: 53,852

Nephritis, nephrotic syndrome, and nephrosis: 39,480

Septicemia: 32,238

(Source: Deuths: Final Data for 2001
http://www.cdc.gov/nchs/fastats/../../data/nvsr/nvsr52/
nvsr52_03.pdf

These statistics don't include the lack of oxygen factors for the first three causes of death — a HUGE issue related to breathing! Your best source of oxygen is the way you breathe so MAKE THE WAY YOU BREATHE YOUR FIRST PRIORITY.

Improved Breathing Can Dramatically Influence Your Life Skills in These Ways:

* Increased productivity
* More stamina
* More joy
* Personal power
* Self -awareness
* Sports performance
* Greater enthusiasm
* Greater sense of belonging
* Acting on authentic self
* Comfort with personal expression
* Contribute to your greater good
* Increased self understanding
* Better decision-making
* Greater motivation
* Expanded options
* More comfortable with change
* Releasing mental ruts
* Improved creativity
* Improved inner strength
* Opening to the state of flow
* New concepts readily integrated
* Less Perfectionism
* Being a self-starter
* Peace of Mind
* Focused thinking
* Spiritual growth

* Alignment between inner drives & outer expression

"Breathing is the first place, not the last,
one should look to when fatigue, disease
or other evidence of disordered energy presents itself."

Dr. Sheldon Hendler in *The Oxygen Breakthrough*

☆ Breathing is a skill you need to <u>develop</u>! Regarding the body and its varied functions: it is an age-old fact that if we don't use something we lose it. If we do not use our breathing correctly we will either lose volume, balance or both, and if we develop breathing incorrectly, we will make an incorrect way of breathing permanent. Our UDB check sheet and free breathing tests can alert you to the presence of poor breathing —so you can change your breathing habits and live longer healthier lives.

☆ Did you know that there are many breathing exercises that make your breathing worse, not better? I see this happening time and time again where someone has been trained in an improper breathing exercise(s) has developed UDB that mimics the exercise they practiced! Once improper breathing exercises are "imprinted in the muscle and connective tissue cell's memory," these habits are hard to eliminate unless you use the specific techniques and exercises contained in our Optimal Breathing® System.

ROSETTA STONE: THE STORY OF A KEY

The Rosetta Stone for breathing is the natural, effortless inhale — your breathing reflex.

A slab of black basalt was found in 1799 near the mouth of the Nile River in Egypt. A decree carved in hieroglyphic and demotic ancient Egyptian writing and Greek provided the key to the deciphering of Egyptian hieroglyphics.

Just as the Rosetta Stone was a key to enabling modern people (for the first time) to translate ancient Egyptian language, key breathing development techniques and exercises contained in our **Optimal Breathing® Development System** guided me into simultaneously combined states of increased energy, mental clarity, emotional calm, physical ease, and balanced breathing freedom. This new way of breathing helped re-establish breathing awareness and internal coordination that had eluded me for over forty years!

☆ Did you know that many people hold their breath and don't even know it? This largely stems from childhood. Being stressed causes us to hold in our belly muscles. Science calls this reaction the "startle reflex." Done often enough in the formative years of childhood causes permanent restrictions or breath holding habits that never go away. Some develop a tendency towards breath holding that is not obvious but reappears during stressful adulthood. Many aspects of shortness of breath appear later in life and are often called (or misnamed) "asthma." The cause of shortness of breath is a <u>mechanical breathing issue</u> that we call Undetected or **Unbalanced Dysfunctional Breathing** or **UDB**.

The Natural Breathing Reflex, like the Rosetta Stone, is a "Key."
It can be developed, along with an improved sensory awareness.

"The Breathing Reflex" is at the bottom of the exhale and immediately following the pause (there <u>should</u> be a pause!). There is a natural autonomic reflex that is triggered to

16

"breathe the body," so to speak. The Breathing Reflex is, or becomes, a "non-pulled-in" inhale that occurs when the body "decides" it needs more oxygen and for nervous system balance. It can be triggered/induced or completely passive depending on the state of body oxygen, depths of rest, or release of tensions needed for recovery of energy and nervous system balance. The Breathing Reflex is addressed throughout the *Secrets* manual, videos and recorded exercises to assist your discovery and development. (Please note that much of breathing awareness must be addressed via a video or audio guide to have any real depth of meaning.) Reading about breathing is helpful and lends deeper insights, but your breathing MUST be properly guided and deeply experienced to be accurately learned and not develop unbalanced or dysfunctional breathing habits.

☆ Did you know that pain increases as breathing quality deteriorates... and dehydration increases as well? We do not get old as much as we dry out. Our cells do not hydrate as they get weaker. Your lungs use a quart of water per day to keep their mucous membranes adequately moisturized!
(http://www.breathing.com/watercure.htm).

☆ Did you know that when you breathe right — you can sing? Human sound is caused as wind passes membranes, muscles, tendons and bones, while creating friction and vibration. Singing is mostly about vibration. Even deaf people can sing. They can be trained to feel the *vibrations* on an acoustic piano and make the sounds they feel from their fingers and hands. Everyone has the potential to sing, but most people do not breathe well and because of that they never learn to sing well, or at all.

ENVIRONMENT

✰ Aside from poor air quality and a toxic environment, do you know that how you sit can dramatically affect your breathing! Posture is critical to optimal breathing. If the body is bent forward — even the slightest — the diaphragm can't rise enough to be able to draw in sufficient air to energize the body.

Do you too often go to sleep watching a TV program or the theater, symphony or movies — when you wish you'd stayed awake to see the event? The culprits are most likely your easy chair or theater seat, posture and the way they make you breathe.

✰ Did you know that belly breathing is not optimal breathing? Look at your entire breathing dynamic to see what is needed. The belly is merely a part of the breathing cycle. Call it an arc, or part of a circle. This circle includes your belly, sides and back for **Optimal Breathing®**. The breathing cycle is round. The diaphragm is round. The lungs are round. Your thorax is round. Breathing must be from the belly, front, sides, and back of your lower, mid and upper trunk to be optimal. Sequencing between these dozens of chambers and compartment needs also to be smooth and balanced .

ANXIETY?

✰ Did you know that (excluding incidences of anxiety caused by stimulants or harmful prescription drugs) most aspects of anxiety and panic attacks can be neutralized with Optimal Breathing®? The way you breathe drives your nervous system — somewhere between the way a 3-year-old child would drive the family car, verses the way a race car driver

18

skillfully navigates through a high speed race! Panic is at one end and relaxation and control are at the opposite end of proper breathing.

SLEEP PROBLEMS?

☆ Did you know that the way you breathe during waking hours carries over into sleep. It works BOTH ways. Bad breathing makes sleep problematic. Great breathing makes sleep better and more restful. Simple as that.

DO YOU KNOW THAT HEADACHES OFTEN STEM FROM POORLY BALANCED BREATHING?

Toxins and allergies not withstanding, ever know someone to BLOW THEIR TOP or get very angry? Remember doing a hand or headstand and how the blood rushes to your head and causes a pressure sensation?

The way the nervous system is driven by uncontrolled excessive high chest breathing causes similar pressure to travel upward into the neck, shoulders and head. So when someone gets afraid or angry, the pressure caused by your body's reaction to that anger travels upward into the closed system of the skull and the brain gets overwhelmed. and This causes the excessive pressure we know as a "headache". Strokes and high blood pressure are often caused or made worsen by this upward pressure.

STRESS?

Most stress is related to poor choices and improper breathing. I once told a client I could train him to walk calmly through the gates of Hell. He replied with a wry smile that walking into Hell was not on his agenda. But we DO on occasion have days from Hell, don't we? Wouldn't it be great to neutralize stress(es) the moment it/they occurred, or have non-drug and no-alcohol ways of rapidly recovering from stress?

Once your breathing skills run more of the show (or better drives the hyopthetical car) your choices become wiser and more clearly defined.

HOT FLASHES ARE OFTEN REDUCED OR ELIMINATED BY PROPER BREATHING!

Along with ALL other body systems, hormonal fluctuations are often driven by an erratic nervous system. Think of this as stress causing the weakest or most vulnerable body system to begin to break down.

EYESIGHT

☆ Did you know that improved breathing will often improve vision? One of our breathing development trainers had a client read an eye chart before an Optimal Breathing Session. Just one session enabled the client to read a smaller line on the eye chart.

NO ONE REALIZED THEY HAD POOR BREATHING!

I read about medical students who simply watched breathing patterns in the waiting room of a doctor's office. They observed that nearly **84 percent** of the people in the waiting room had disturbed breathing patterns, indicating potential **Unbalanced Deep Breathing** (see UDB evaluation). The article went on to say that regardless of their medical problem, more than 2/3 of those patients seemed to have disturbed breathing! The author commented that none of those people were there to find out how to <u>improve</u> their breathing.

BREATHING DEVELOPMENT AS A PRIMARY GOAL INSTEAD OF AN AFTERTHOUGHT.

Though breathing exercises are no guarantee of optimal breathing, Doctors Dean Ornish, Andrew Weil, Len Saputo, Sheldon Hendler and Gabriel Cousens all highly recommend exercises. The only questions are "which ones"?

History has many examples of using breathing to augment other systems of health and personal power. (There are at least 5,000 published papers on influences on the way people breathe) but to the best of our knowledge the idea of making breathing the primary focus has not been explored until the **Optimal Breathing System**[a].

Singing, chanting and toning have been health, personal and spiritual growth tools for thousands of years! The only question is which exercises are more appropriate, harmful, confusing or pretty much a waste of time, depending on the goal(s) of the individual..

With thousands of voice teachers, more than 2,400 varieties of Chinese Qi Gong (chi kung) and other ways of manipulating the life-force (chi), plus the Hindu school of pranayama that is rapidly entering mainstream scientific consciousness, we have choices that may be great or not so great.

At present there is NO leading role model for what's "*best*," though colleagues of mine are addressing this issue. My one caution in this area is you need to know that breathing exercises, done repeatedly without professional and accountable guidance, may well *distort* healthy breathing patterns and sequencing.

The bottom line is that all of us need some manner of breathing trainer/coach to learn to breathe optimally. We can often progress on our own and get significant, even life saving benefits, but eventually we need an experienced human to give us moment-to-moment feedback on whether we are properly performing good to great breathing.

Did you know you can raise your oxygen levels without exercise?

Proper exercise is wonderful but many people can not or do not have the energy to exercise.

A key factor is raising the natural oxygen levels — without exercise — is to breathe in a certain way more than you need, without moving, which uses up the oxygen reserve. Our *Better Breathing Exercise #2* is great for this!

INTRODUCING THE NEED FOR DETOXIFICATION

Your skin and the way you breathe are the biggest detoxification systems in your body! How well couples breathe greatly affects the quality of the eggs and sperm they produce, thus influencing the quality and genetic make-up of their prospective child. Poor breathing moves few, if any toxins out of the body, especially the lungs, and can cause back ups in many detoxification systems in the body.

Researchers at Duke University in North Carolina learned what mothers eat and drink during pregnancy has a fundamental and lifelong affect on the genes of their children and their children's children!

These researchers found they could change the coat color of baby mice by feeding their mothers different levels of nutrients during pregnancy, which altered how the pups' cells read their genes. The nutritionally-supplemented mice were less prone to obesity and diabetes than genetically identical mice whose mothers received no supplement.

It makes sense to assume that proper nutrition in humans could impact even more important changes to offspring, since human genes are much more complex than mice.

Breathing would be THE major factor affected by improper water, nutrition and toxins when the DNA is genetically-challenged.

Mutation changes the DNA, the sequencing of genes, but research proved that genetic and nutritional factors can alter how a gene is used, while leaving the DNA sequence unchanged. (For more about this go to **www.newscientist.com** or www.google.com and type "*mother at*e" in the search engine). This supports the research of Linus Pauling, George Watson, Earl Mindell and thousands of clinical nutritionists who support nutritional supplementation to maintain proper health balance. Learn more about all this in ***Building Healthy Lungs, Naturally***.

YOUR PAST AND PRESENT

You are also the product of your parents and ancestors and how all of them lived. Put all of this together and evaluate who YOU are NOW.

We all can make changes to improve our health. Lets look at the various parts that comprise the whole we call "me" ... and how breathing can be affected.

Profession

Are you active in your work? Do you play sports, indoors or out? Do you farm, build roads or bridges, chase after your young children all day, or physically move about in your work?

Or, do you sit at a desk inside a closed office all day and your physical activity is limited? Is your posture and deep breathing limited and your access to fresh air reduced?

(Learn more about all of this in *Secrets of Optimal Natural Breathing Development & Building Healthy Lungs, Naturally.*)

Lifestyle

Are you a quiet, introverted person... or are you the opposite - the life of the party?

Did you overeat? Do you eat healthy foods and drink lots of water? Do you exercise? Do you smoke? Do you drink alcohol? Too much? Too often?

Did you live in a clean environment, or are your skies filled with smog and pollutants? Is your water and land clean or environmentally hazardous to your health?

Once we see the greater picture of who we actually are, we get a better understanding of the good and the bad aspects of the "me" that we have become.

The next step is to begin changing the bad/unhealthy aspects so they are no longer detrimental to your health and well-being.

(Learn more about all of this in *Secrets of Optimal Natural Breathing Development & Building Healthy Lungs, Naturally.*)

Our Parents

Check out Mom and Dad. Were either of them overweight? Did they eat properly? Did they drink adequate amounts of water? Did they exercise? Did they smoke? Are or were they healthy emotionally? Did you know that most, if not all emotionally related issues including phobias have a significant breathing-related issue. Did they sing or hum a lot to themselves or others? These are simple habits that seem to calm and resolve many daily stresses and challenges to daily modern living.

What were their professions? Did they receive good non-drug oriented health care and counseling? .Probably not. Chances are some of these areas are very suspect. After all, times have certainly changed! We now know more about nutrition and exercise and their benefits to a healthier body and lifestyle than our parents knew.

Part of this new knowledge is the result of our own un-doing.

We've polluted our ground and streams, so we have to study these problems in order to fix them — and to fix ourselves. We've also changed from a rural, agrarian lifestyle to (mostly) sitting inside our offices most of the day. All of this adds to our health challenges.

Our grandparents and parents may have been more inclined towards fatty meals to sustain them during a long farming day.

With the broad use of the automobile, they became more inclined to drive instead of walking. With the expansion of travel they came into contact with people from other geographical areas and countries, possibly adding parasites and disease and the affects to their genes.

We like to imitate our parents, our role models. So we are likely to pick up their habits, both good and bad.

Pregnancy

"Did you know that the size of the fetus in the third trimester causes breathing restrictions and CO_2/O_2 imbalances in the mother's blood supply and subsequent reduced blood flow to the placenta? This causes an increase

in breathing rate and progesterone. This invites sustained loss of magnesium begetting convulsions and cramps"
— Dr. Peter Litchfield

While your mother was pregnant with you, did she have good, healthy habits? Did she eat proper foods, drink enough water, eliminate smoking and alcohol well PRIOR to getting pregnant, get regular medical check-ups, rest and exercise, stay in balance emotionally?

Emotions and breathing are interdependent and effect each other as much as water effects thirst and vice versa. (Learn more in *Secrets of Optimal Natural Breathing Development & Building Healthy Lungs, Naturally.*)

Genetics

The genetic make-up of our ancestors helped define who we are. The good and bad genes pass on certain strengths and weaknesses. One person may have large lungs and a small breathing passageway or the reverse. One may be tall and thin with large or small lungs or diaphragm, while another is short and stout with small or large lungs or diaphragm. Another may inherit asthma-like symptoms. Another (only a VERY small percentage) have some sort of genetic deficiency.

I believe, in general, that genetic makeup or predisposition are highly overrated and the individual has more to say about how they evolve then the geneticists want us to believe. Read more abut this in *Unstoppable* by Cynthia Kersey (see **Resources** section). You can also learn about a young man who was born with no arms.

Knowledge, natural hygiene and faith in one's higher power are powerful factors that often make genetics seem puny by comparison. You simply must learn what factors are more relevant to your goals and purposes.

To reduce the possibility that negative genes are gong to dominate, regardless of what childbearing-age people do, they should focus on building healthy genes before conception. That means taking care of themselves NOW.

Worldwide, sperm counts are dropping and egg quality has declined

Many factors can affect the number, strength and vitality of sperm and eggs and even the genetic material they carry. For many reasons, men's sperm counts worldwide have been dropping over the last 50 years. Toxins in and EMFs (electrical magnetic frequencies – cell towers and power lines) damage sperm and egg quality and cause a myriad of health challenges. Smoking, sexually transmitted diseases and especially environmental toxins (including personal care and cleaning products) are making men and women sterile. Both parents exposure to chemicals also increases the risk of miscarriage. . (To learn more on a regular basis, send an email to: *eSens-subscribe@yahoo groups.com*, plus check out *Body Burden* at this website: http://*www.ewg.org*.

Parents who smoke are more likely to have children with a cleft lip and palate. Both cigarette smoking and alcohol use by prospective parents increases the risk of the baby's having a heart defect and breathing problems.

You are what your mother and father ate and drank and the way - and the quality of air - they breathed!

Couples of child-bearing age who are willing to focus on their future children's health, rather than on their own desires, should significantly improve their own health, thus producing healthier genetic materials to produce a healthier child(ren).

Whether male or female, we suggest you view all dietary

and water (H_20 = hydrogen and oxygen) decisions from the perspective that you could get pregnant and need to be thinking about how your diet (including cleansings) are impacting the fetus — your children and their children's future!

DON'T PUT THAT TOXIC DEAD THING IN YOUR MOUTH!

Remember the ad that jokingly suggested to "Give it to Mikey, he'll eat anything"?
Even a joking suggestion like that gives the wrong impression about the importance of what we eat.

"Proper nutrition" means eliminating foods and drinks that provide <u>no</u> nutrition, enzymes or energy, are toxic, or difficult to digest.

The offending foods that most consume:
Dairy products - pasteurized and homogenized. (non-raw)
http://www.breathing.com/articles/not-milk.htm
Sugar and most sugar substitutes (Stevia is OK to use)
http://www.breathing.com/sugar-124ways.htm
Sodas & soft drinks
http://www.breathing.com/articles/soda-pop-dangers.htm
   Trust me. Drinking carbonated beverages is NOT a good thing to do.
   <u>The carbonation replaces oxygen in your body</u>!
   It takes 2 GALLONS of water to neutralize the acid in one soda!

(http://*www.breathing.com/articles/watercure.htm*)

Breads, pastries, cereals, cookies and other refined grain products (wheat, rye, barley)
É anything containing white flour and sugar
http://www.breathing.com/grain-damage.htm
Margarine (it's ONE molecule away from being plastic!)
Hydrogenated vegetable oils (a major cause of macular degeneration & heart problems)
http://www.breathing.com/articles/macular-degeneration.htm
Canned or frozen anything
Microwaved foods. *http://breathing.com/articles/ microwaves.htm*
Too many cooked foods.
Non-organic anything.

☆ Do you know that poor breathing can cause blood acidosis or respiratory alkalosis, either of which will compromise cellular function and/or oxygen transfer into your cells and hemoglobin?

WHAT ELSE?

So now you know you are what you eat and drink — at any age! Proper nutrition and water and detoxification helps the cells replace and multiply. Without this, the lungs have to divert much of their natural healing and rebuilding powers to repairing and eliminating toxins, caused by insufficient cellular activity.

☆ Do you know your entire body is regenerated over a seven (7) year period, even your teeth and bones! A fetus' cells are replicating in the millions per day. So what your mother ate and her emotional state as well as cellular oxygen levels is critical to your current health.

Many other interesting facts about the way you breathe are

more fully explained in my *Secrets of Optimal Breathing Development* and in *Building Healthy Lungs, Naturally*.

Meanwhile consider the following:.
1. Over 90% of your energy should come from your breathing.
2. Clinical studies prove that oxygen, wellness and sickness are totally dependent upon the way we breathe and oxygenate our system.
3. Bad breathing can make your blood too acidic adversely effecting EVERY critical cellular action.
4. Aerobics can have short-term benefits and long term harm to your breathing
5. So called altitude sickness may be partially or completely eliminated with proper breathing.
6. Blood carbon dioxide levels are often too low causing poorly oxygenated brain and organ systems.
7. The way you breathe is the best stress manager (better than living on a private deserted island!)
8. Arthritis is made worse or improved by the way you breathe
9. Exercise-induced asthma and shortness of breath is often caused by poor breathing.
10. A smooth running nervous system requires smooth and balanced breathing
11. Pregnancy is harmful to breathing, especially in the third trimester
12. Poor maternal prenatal breathing often causes insufficient nutrients to the placenta
13. Your breathing can be coordinated, but still be shallow
14. Breathing deeper often causes breathing restrictions
15. Caffeine destroys oxygen, replacing energy with synthetic stimulation

16 Easy natural, effortless breathing is impossible without proper breathing.

17. Everyone can learn to breathe better

18. Most of your lung volume is in your back!

19. Sunken chests and irregularly shaped rib cages can be reformed

20. If your breathing feels like a series of events, instead of one thing, you have a breathing mechanics problem

21. Being overweight restricts breathing, adding to weight gain. (Stress is very acidic and your body needs to be alkaline to stay healthy. Disease can only develop when the body is too acidic ...!)

22. Mind chatter often stems from improper breathing.

23. Washboard abs restrict optimal breathing

24. Speech problems stem largely from UDB

25. Depression can often be relieved by proper breathing

26. Seizures have a huge breathing/UDB component

27. Many breathing-related issues have emotional factors

28. Nightmares are often caused by unresolved emotional issues that are locked in the body's cellular memories by UDB (Unbalanced Dysfunctional Breathing).

29. Negative emotions will dissipate with proper breathing. (UDB causes negative emotions!)

30. Loss of natural teeth (replaced by false or no teeth) can cause up to 85% loss of chewing effectiveness. This places a huge load on the lungs to rid themselves of undigested cellular debris, causing excessive mucous and food allergies that adversely effect lung function.

LEARNING CHALLENGES.

Oxygen concentration and glucose supply in the brain can be reduced by 50% through decreased blood flow via CO_2 deficit and vaso-constriction caused by UDB and CO_2 deficit.

"Blood alkalosis means that hemoglobin is less inclined to distribute oxygen actually present in the brain. Thus, together the net effect of reduced blood flow and disinclined hemoglobin is major reduction in oxygen supply. This 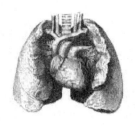 dramatic shift in chemistry can result in the following kinds of performance decrements: **cognitive deficits:** attention, memory, thinking, problem solving, concentrating, multitasking, and judgment. Consider, for example, the impact on attention deficit disorder (ADD) in children and adults." — Dr. Peter Litchfield (see Optimal Breathing® Core Faculty — page 43)

IF YOU WANT TO BE REALLY ALIVE AT AGE 105 YOU NEED TO LEARN TO BREATHE BETTER — TODAY!!

Do not wait until you experience shortness of breath. By then you have probably lost over half your breathing volume. Act now. Results from over 40,000 **Free Breathing Tests**, taken online at ***http://www.breathing.com/tests.htm***, have given us tremendous insights about what is needed to develop your breathing and give you the best odds for having a longer, healthier, more productive and vibrant life.

We guarantee rapid improvement. You have everything to gain and most likely these to lose: health challenges and/or unrealized personal goals.

Take yourself to a higher level by ordering our **#176 Fundamentals of Breathing Development** DVD or video and the **#191 Secrets of Optimal Natural Breathing Development** manual, especially if you'd like to add a new dimension to your health care practice, or perhaps even become an Optimal Breathing® Development Specialist (OBDS).

http://www.breathing.com/school/main.htm

MIKE'S FAVORITE BREATHING EXERCISE
The Squeeze and Breathe® Technique

© 2004 All rights reserved.

http://www.breathing.com/squeezeandbreathe.htm

There are many breathing exercises. For most people, there may be only *one* really good exercise that works *well* as a starting point to guide someone with poor to very poor breathing. The best exercise(es) either energize or slow down/ calm the breathing, or both. What's *optimal* also increases breathing volume and therefore one's longevity.

The following breathing exercise will help do ALL three: slowing, energizing and expanding. Good endorphin production seems to stem from a strong parasympathetic/ relaxing breathing pattern. When done properly, this exercise increases significant energy, as well as relaxation.

Anxiety can be caused (or stress increased) by poor breathing speed and erratic/unbalanced sequencing. This exercise is very good for reducing anxiety and/or depression. Extreme forms of emotion are often immobilizing, limiting and dangerous to one's health and well-being. Emotions can be deadly. Anxiety can harm and even kill. The way you breathe can reduce or increase your emotional/fear response.

Look at the lungs above (cut back to show how the heart fits into that space). Notice how the lungs are smaller at the top. This means it's pointless to breathe into the high chest because there's very little lung volume there.

The mid chest and lower rear lung lobes are where the major breathing volume is obtained (the back of the trunk from

33

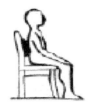

mid back to waist). This area allows the most expansion. Tension in the low back tends to restrict expansion, so we must both access and challenge that area in the following way.

For breathing that is quieting, calming, centering and energizing all at once: Stand with knees slightly bent is preferable with tail bone tilted gently forward.

Or

Supported by a small round pillow (at left) or use a NADA Chair (on right), http://www.breathing.com/nada.htm sit near the front edge of a fairly hard surfaced chair, stool or arm of a couch, with your feet flat on the floor. Both of these positions need an erect but not stiff posture. Stand or sit "tallest" with your chin even with (or above) the horizon and gently tucked in.

If you stand, bend your knees slightly to unlock them.

Lightly touch your tongue to the roof of your mouth and let your jaw relax. Relax your belly. Let it hang down. Let go of any thought of having a "pot belly" or not having "washboard abs".

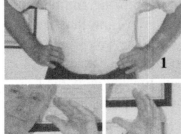

Place your thumbs over your kidneys (below your back ribs and above your pelvis - (photo #1 at left). Wrap your fingers around your sides towards your belly button (as if you are getting a front-to-back firm grip on "love handles" - or that general area). Get a good grip by squeezing your fingers and

thumbs together firmly, then breathe through your nose (a long, slow, deep 3-count in-breath). Force your squeezed fingers (Photo #2) apart with your in-breath, against the tension in your squeezed fingers. (Use the force of breathing-in to make your fingers and thumbs expand.)

Then relax your grip (Photo #3) and slow down the exhale so it lasts for a count of seven (7). Never tighten the belly to extend the exhale. Simply slow the speed of the out-breath. Always keep the belly relaxed.

Do this exercise again, use a 3-count inhale and 7-count exhale.

If you did not feel better from this exercise, we encourage you to take our Free Breathing Tests and see why and how to develop your breathing: http://www.breathing.com/tests.htm

HOW DID IT FEEL?

Dizziness, spacey ness, or confusion or anxiety means you:
A. Probably did not squeeze in the right place – like on the bone of the pelvis or ribs or squeeze or did not squeeze hard enough.
B. Or you breathed too fast. SLOW down the exhale by adding 3-7 counts to the exhale and try it again in one minute.
C. You need another try so it's better at it so wait a minute or two, after the energy has subsided or integrated within you and do it again.
D. Still anxious or dizzy or both? - You may have a severe case of UDB - in which case you should stop and call us for a recommendation.
E. You REALLY need to learn this!

It felt relaxing, energizing? Are you calmer? Energized?
Calm and energized at the same time? Anxious? If anxious, try to lengthen the exhale count, while keeping the inhale count the same or smaller. Example: a 3 count inhale and 10 count exhale or 3 count inhale and 12 count exhale. A 20 count exhale should eventually be attainable, but for some people it might take weeks or months to develop. (Remember: NEVER tighten your belly to make the exhale last longer.) Just let the air out slower. You should eventually feel a calming and energizing effect throughout your entire body.

If that is not the right feel or timing, then experiment with the same inhales, but longer or shorter exhales, until you discover a comfortable pattern that you can repeat .

The Squeeze & Breathe Technique® is very powerful, but is still a temporary approach. If it helps you stay calm or energized, even just a little bit, I urge you to take it to the higher and higher levels for your maximum health maintenance. (Recommended: *#176 DVD/video Fundamentals* Program
http://www.breathing.com/video-strap.htm)

Use our comprehensive way of evaluating your breathing! take our FREE BREATHING TESTS at
http://www.breathing.com/tests.htm

Chapter 2
What are the Obstacles to Optimal Breathing?
Are You Among Those Considered at "High Risk" of Oxygen Deficiency?

"Insufficient oxygen means insufficient biological energy that can result in anything from mild fatigue to life-threatening disease. The link between insufficient oxygen and disease has now been firmly established."
— Dr. W. Spencer Way in the ***Journal of American Association of Physicians***

Oxygen Deficiency is Often Overlooked As A Cause for Symptoms of:

Acid Stomach
Addictions
Allergies
Anger or Sadness
Anxiety, panic, hostility
Asthma
Bacterial, viral & parasite infection
    (including cancer)
Bad memory
Cancer
Chest pains

Circulation problems
Depression
Digestive Disorders
Dizziness
Drowsiness
Excessive colds & infections
Exhaustion
Fatigue
Forgetfulness/forgets to breathe
Heart palpitations
Headaches
High blood pressure
Holding breath
Inflamed, swollen or aching joints
Low/No sex drive
Memory loss
Muscle or tendon aches
Overweight
Panic attacks
Phobias
Poor voice quality
Premature aging
Shortness of breath
Skin disorders
Sleeping disorders
Stress/stressed out
Trouble sleeping
Weakened immune system

Researchers have found that besides people with specific oxygen-deficient related health problems, those who live in certain areas, or work in certain occupations or under certain conditions, are more at risk of becoming oxygen-depleted:

- **Elderly**
- **Smokers**
- **Participate in regular heavy exercise**
- **Participate in sports activities**
- **Work in a sealed building**
- **Work in high-stress environments**
- **Work regular excessive hours**
- **Live in cities with high pollution**
- **Live at high altitudes**
    (less oxygen in atmosphere)
- **Frequent airplane flyers**
    (airplane cabins are low in oxygen)
- **Frequent travel across time zones**
- **Frequent work schedule changes from days to nights**

MAJOR MEASURABLE CHALLENGES TO DEVELOPING OPTIMAL BREATHING®

Not necessarily in order of importance
1. Congenital deformity
2. Poor posture
3. Breathing volume
4. Poor nutrition

5. Cellular strength
6. Environmental and food toxicity
7. Lack of physical movement
8. Insufficient water intake
9. Insufficient blood carbon dioxide balance
10. Poor ergonomics
11. Trauma: past, present and the perception of
12. Poor attitude
13. No spiritual life.

OBESITY AND BREATHING

An article entitled *"Effects of Obesity on Respiratory Resistance"* (increased force required to breathe and shortness of breath) in **Chest** magazine, May 1993,103(5):1470-1476, reported findings that suggest *"in addition to the elastic load, obese subjects have to overcome increased respiratory resistance from the reduction in lung volume related to being overweight."*

Weight-loss experts have a novel prescription for people who want to shed pounds: Get some sleep!
http://www.breathing.com/sleep-obesity.com

MYTHS & CAUTIONS ABOUT BREATHING

Breathing Myths

1. Underbreathing is better. Asthma symptoms are because we breathe too much???. A style of asthma reduction advises people to under-breathe. It actually can help reduce asthma symptoms, but I believe this is not optimal as its advocates state that CO_2 is more important than oxygen. The key to relieving or reducing asthma is not volume. It's breathing balance. A shallow chest breath isn't sufficient. People with asthma require a strong belly breath to maintain nervous system balance. Food allergies can be critical as well, but the mechanics of breathing can be changed a lot faster and in conjunction with the diet. (Learn more about this at my website: http://www.breathing.com/articles/buteyko.htm)

2. Oxygen used to be 30-40% of the air we breathe? According to researchers at the Scripps Institute, that's not accurate. Air bubble samples taken from 10,000-year -old icebergs have a few thousands of a percentage more oxygen, but that's all. Oxygen levels are low in many cities with sick buildings and pollution that displaces oxygen levels down to way less than what's healthy and necessary for us today.

3. All breathing exercises are good for you. "I never met a breathing exercise I did not like" was shared with me by an acquaintance who advertises himself as a breathing master. What he later learned is that practice makes permanent, but not necessarily anything close to perfect.

4. Deep breathing is always better. Forced deep breathing can restrict easier, larger deep breathing. For this reason we don't recommend it unless you are in a race or being chased by a wild animal or having great sex!
Healthy deep breathing must be well balanced, with the majority of the lung expansion in the lower front, sides and back of the trunk.

5. Stronger diaphragms are best. Larger is the key word for a diaphragm. If a diaphragm is larger , it should be stronger, but if it is stronger it will not necessarily be larger. Larger begets a higher rise up into the chest and increased volume for better oxygenation and ease of breathing during waking and sleep. Stronger diaphragm begets stronger voice, but perhaps not very much breath/vital capacity.

Breathing Cautions

1. Pranayama is largely for altered states of consciousness. I recommend that if you are going to experiment in pranayama, first develop a strong balanced breath so your nervous system knows *where* to revert to after the altered -state experience, so you know where "home base" is located and what it "feels like." Pranayama needs an experienced teacher with adequate credentials to teach it. (Learn more about Pranayama here:
http://www.breathing.com/articles/pranayama.htm)

2. Oxygen bars are a huge waste of money (in my opinion), compared to hyberbaric oxygen tank treatments at two atmospheres of pressure. I suspect it would take tens of thousands of dollars of sniffing oxygen from a bottle to get even a small percentage of the benefits of one $100 hyperbaric chamber treatment. Oxygen bars are nice places to meet like-minded health conscious people and learn to appreciate oxygen even more, but for breathing and oxygen saturation to aid a health issue and act as a significant preventive, I suggest you learn to breathe better and get as much as you can for free!

3. Confusion abounds about hyperbaric oxygen tanks. Beware of inexpensive hyperbaric oxygen tank substitutes that use little to no atmospheric pressure and still call themselves hyperbaric. They just leave out the oxygen part. Hmmmm. They are often beneficial, but not nearly as effective as the highly pressurized hyperbaric

chambers. (Learn more here: ***http://www.breathing.com/articles/
hyperberic.htm***   See ***http://www.miraclemountain.org*** for a cost-
effective source.)

Use our comprehensive way of evaluating your breathing!
Take our FREE BREATHING TESTS at
http://www.breathing.com/tests.htm

Chapter 3
OVERCOMING THE OBSTACLES BEGINS WITH FULLY APPRECIATING THE POSSIBILITIES

MOMENT TO MOMENT EXPERIENCES THAT INDICATE AVERAGE TO GOOD TO GREAT BREATHING

1. Open, free, easy breathing in chest, sides, back, belly
2. Nostrils open and free
3. Never sick
4. Wake up refreshed
5. Steady to great energy throughout the day
6. Quick recovery from physical exertion or stress
7. Good mood, positive can-do attitude
8. Clear-headed
9. Strong and free self expression
10. Strong self esteem
11. Healthy relationships (5 or more)
12. Breathing changes when communicating with loved ones about specific issues — which you resolve positively
13. Breathing changes around specific people, places or things — and you stay positive

Learn How Optimal Breathing® Can Improve Your Health & Life

IMMUNE SYSTEM

- Although it's not thought of that way, oxygen really is a primary component of the immune system. People often die in hospitals from a combination of pneumonia and immune system weakness.
- Oxygen levels, breathing and the immune system are completely inter-dependent.

Your breath and breathing aids your immune system in these ways:

- Lessens stress responses by regulating the nervous system that staves off diverting energy from healthy immune system function while increasing oxygen to kill germs, viruses and parasites and support healthy bacteria. .
- Oxygen works very much like T-cells as it kills harmful bacteria, germs and viruses.
- Increasing oxygen offsets fatigue, listlessness, repeated infections, inflammations, allergic reactions, slow wound healing, chronic diarrhea and infections that represent an overgrowth of some normally present organism, such as oral thrush, systemic Candida or vaginal yeast infections.
- Better breathing supplies extra oxygen molecules that attach to toxins and pollution and form toxic waste that is excreted from the body via the breath and other means of elimination which reduces the work of the immune system.
- Accelerating regeneration of tissues by allowing the regenerative systems of the body to heal/regenerate instead of fight off invaders.

45

THE RESPIRATORY SYSTEM

- Dramatically aids in relief of many long term respiratory difficulties such as asthma, bronchitis, COPD
- Optimal Breathing® can reduce chest pains due to tight muscles, thus the tension -causing anxiety of "heart attack potential" is reduced. For example: the strapping/belt technique opens up the chest and allows the chest, belly, back and sides to communicate simultaneously laterally, right to left, as well as from front to back. When one progresses from up to down, all 3 planes, syncrhythmically together, and the primitive reflexes that connect to the breathing are able to reconnect, sequence and balance.
- Opens up the chest to make breathing easier and fuller, which facilitates strengthening of the life force, emotional stability and mental clarity to feel more energetic.
- Maintains blood acid/alkaline balance which supports optimal cellular function

CIRCULATORY SYSTEM

- Improves blood circulation and relieves congestion
- Increases supply of oxygen and nutrients to cells throughout the body
- Increases flow of oxygen-to-oxygen loving organs such as the brain and eyes
- Eases the strain on the heart by increasing oxygen to the heart

THE NERVOUS SYSTEM

- Calms a chronic "fright or flight" anxiety state by reversing the breathing patterns which began at the time of the original trauma
- Healthfully stimulates the nervous system when fatigue is present

46

- Helps reduce overeating response to stress
- Depending on the technique used, healthy breathing can balance brain hemispheres

THE DIGESTIVE SYSTEM
- Proper diaphragmatic action acts as a pump to massage the internal organs, significantly aiding their function
- Optimal breathing calms the emotions which in turn allow the digestive system to stay in a stronger expression of parasympathetic rest, digest and heal.

URINARY SYSTEM
- Excess water (in the form of vapor) is expelled
- Reduces swelling of the body (edema)
- Decreases stress on organs of elimination, thus helping the body to naturally cleanse and tonify

THE LYMPHATIC SYSTEM
- Increases depth and continuity of lymphatic fluid circulation, which plays a crucial role in eliminating toxic waste and strengthening the immune system
- Helps speed recovery after major illnesses

MUSCLES/LIGAMENTS
- Relaxes muscle spasm and relieves tension. Tension that often causes muscle weakness
- Helps increase the supply of blood and nutrients to muscle
- Upper body strength is directly affected by proper breathing
- Feeling better and more "present" in your body naturally leads to a greater desire to exercise for health and enjoyment
- Offsets and prevents formation of adhesions

- Improves coordination and grace via greater relaxation and self-awareness

STRUCTURAL
- Moment to moment 24-7-365 fluidity of all movement whether walking, running, swimming, dancing or crawling.
- Invites internal sensing of optimal posturing
- Helps prevent muscle adhesions
- Releases and reduces muscular tension that eventually may cause structural problems
- Helps increase flexibility and strength of joints; when you breathe easier you move easier
- Can partially compensate for lack of exercise and inactivity due to habit, illness or injury

ATHLETIC PERFORMANCE
- Enhance endurance
- Shorten recovery times.
- Smooth out running styles, creating grace, ease and more efficient movement
- Sharpen mental clarity

PHYSICAL APPEARANCE
- Healthy breathing helps you look more rested and vibrant
- Reduces wrinkles due to improved circulation and blood oxygen flow
- Results in radiant skin at any age
- Replaces energy lost during the natural process of growth and aging
- You smile more

MENTAL
- Improves power of mental concentration and observation
- The brain is an oxygen-loving organ; I've often read where it uses up to 40% of our O2 supply.
- Lower stress levels lead to higher productivity, greater learning capacity, better decision making

EMOTIONAL
- Increases feelings of safety, nurturing and self-acceptance
- Produces profound relaxation and inner peace (think: grace under pressure and courage under fire)
- Reverses effects of stress related to self-defeating habits and tendencies, including childhood traumas, religious programming and cultural conditioning
- Strengthens coping skills
- Increases positive energy
- Enhances sense of self and inner power
- Produces heightened self-awareness and self-love, which leads to healthier life choices about self-care, relationships, work, environment, etc.

SPIRITUAL
- Deepens meditation or spiritual connection
- Heightens intuition
- Balances subtle energy systems affecting all the bodies: physical, emotional, mental, spiritual
- Enhances creativity

INTERPERSONAL RELATIONSHIPS
- Relaxation, self-love and self-acceptance enhanced by optimal

breathing leads to greater compassion for others
- Helps clarify and strengthen boundaries and take responsibility for their role in relationships
- Increases awareness and management of subtle energies within and around you and others

SEXUAL ENJOYMENT
- Regulates intensity of orgasm
- Higher relaxation levels and self-love lead to more compatible partner choices

PRODUCTIVITY
- Feel more rested and get more done.

These are some OPTIMAL VITALITY GOALS©

Check (✔) the ones you want to improve.

(If you have suggestions for additional goals, please send them to mw@breathing.com)

Put "My Optimal Vitality Goals" in the SUBJECT line.

- ☆ Improve my diet
- ☆ Drink 4 quarts water daily
- ☆ Increased productivity
- ☆ More stamina
- ☆ More joy
- ☆ Personal power
- ☆ Self -awareness
- ☆ Sports performance
- ☆ Greater enthusiasm
- ☆ Greater sense of belonging
- ☆ Acting on authentic self
- ☆ Comfort with personal expression
- ☆ Contribute to your greater good
- ☆ Increased self understanding
- ☆ Better decision-making
- ☆ Greater motivation
- ☆ Expanded options
- ☆ More comfortable with change
- ☆ Releasing mental ruts
- ☆ Improved creativity
- ☆ Improved inner strength
- ☆ Opening to the state of flow
- ☆ New concepts readily integrated
- ☆ Less Perfectionism
- ☆ Being a self-starter
- ☆ Peace of Mind
- ☆ Focused thinking
- ☆ Spiritual growth
- ☆ Alignment between inner drives & outer expression

Your improvements on the **Optimal Vitality Goals**© list (above) are best achieved through our Breathing Development Self-Help Programs found at: **http://www.breathing.com/programs.htm** or through personal trainings with an **Optimal Breathing Development Specialist.** Find an OBDS in your area at this webpage: **http://www.breathing.com/school/refer.htm**

As your scores improve on the following UDB list, your OPTIMAL VITALITY FACTORS should also improve!

HOW MANY AREAS OF YOUR LIFE TODAY ARE AFFECTED BY THE WAY YOU BREATHE?

Circle the number(s) of challenges you presently experience on the UDB list on the next page.
What major issues do you most want to improve? (Circle the whole line.)

At your subsequent evaluations:
  • indicate if your progress is good and you want more,
  • or do you need to change what you're doing?

Use our comprehensive way of evaluating your breathing!
Take our FREE BREATHING TESTS: *http://www.breathing.com/tests.htm*

Unbalanced Dysfunctional Breathing - UDB

UDB causes or increases shortness of breath, hyperventilation, anxiety, panic attacks, seizures, asthma, COPD, nervous system dysfunction, etc. Bad breathing can: *make you anxious *make you sick/sicker *make you think you're crazy *destroy your energy *make/keep you fat *steal your personal power *hinder your voice and *shorten your life. Your breathing may be "authentic" but still severely unbalanced. **Make copies of this page so you can record your progress for 3-6 months.** Or download our PDF file to keep on file.
 http://www.breathing.com/udb.htm Check (✔) the numbers (issues) you're
experiencing <u>now</u>. At subsequent evaluations, report good progress or where you feel you need to improve or change what you're doing. Close your eyes, go within and inhale and exhale deeply (twice), as you would normally breathe. Open your eyes and reflect on whether you (now or often) experience any of these issues. More than two circles means you are experiencing UDB.

Breath is life! *Improve your breathing NOW* !!

1.   Addicted
2.   Air hunger
3.   Allergies
4.   Altitude makes breathing harder
5.   Anger
6.   Anxiety
7.   Apathy

8. Apnea
9. Attention problems
70. Back pain–low or mid back
11. Bluish cast to lips, nail beds
12. Bowel or rectum disorder
13. Blood sugar swings (wide)
14. Look in a mirror and breathe as deeply as you can. Do your neck muscles bulge out? Your shoulders or collar bones rise?
15. Breathing feels like a series of events, instead of one smooth internally coordina ted continuous flow
16. Breathing feels stuck
17. Breath heaving
18. Breathing labored/restricted
19. Breathing is shallow
20. Breathlessness
21. Can't catch breath or deep breathing curtailed
22. Can't feel breath in nostrils
23. Can't meditate
24. Can't relax
25. Can't sleep on back
26. Can't walk and easily talk at the same time
27. Chest is large and stiff
28. Chest pain
29. Chest sunken
30. Chest tightness after surgery

31. Chest wall defects (faults)
32. Chest wall tenderness
33. Chronic cough
34. Chronic pain
35. Cold hands or sweaty palms
36. Cold temp bothers breathing
37. Confrontations make your voice pitch go up
38. Confused or sense of losing normal contact with surroundings
39. Constant Fatigue
40. Constipation
41. Cramps in abdomen or below sternum, or side stitches
42. Depression
43. Digestion poor
44. Diaphragm excursion poor
45. Diaphragmatic impairment
46. Dizzy when excited-anxious
47. Do you often PRESS your tongue to the roof of your mouth?
48. Dry mouth
49. Fanny sticks out in rear
50. Fall asleep watching TV or at theater when you would rather watch program?
51. Feel a hitch, bump or lump right below your breastbone when you try to take a deep breath
52. Feelings of suffocation

53. Finish other people's sentences for them
54. Furrows brow often
55. Gasping
56. Get tired from reading out loud?
57. Get drowsy from driving a vehicle
58. Grind teeth at night
59. Dynamic hyperinflation
60. Headaches
61. Heart condition or attack(s)
62. Heavy breathing
63. High blood pressure
64. History or present lung disease
65. History of abuse or trauma
66. Hold breath a lot
67. Hormonal fluctuations
68. Hot flashes
69. Hyperventilation, overbreathing
70. Hypocapnea (exhale too little carbon dioxide)
71. Hypoglycemia
72. Irregular heartbeats
73. Irregularly formed rib cag (can you see it in mirror?)
74. Jaw tension
75. Jet lag or severe jet lag
76. Longevity wanted
77. Lump in throat
78. Migraines

79. Mouth breather
80. Nightmares
81. Nodules
82. Obese
83. Often catch yourself not breathing?
84. Often shift weight from side to side while standing
85. Panic attacks
85. People have difficulty hearing you and are not partly deaf
86. Phobic
87. Poor boundaries
88. Poor sleep
89. Posture poor
90. Pregnant
91. Public speaking
92. Pulsing or stabbing feeling in and around ribs
93. Reduced pain tolerance
94. Reflux
95. Repetitive strain injury
96. Ribs flair outward at bottom during inhale
97. Sallow complexion
98. Scoliosis or abnormal curvature of the spine
99. Seizures
100. Self Esteem Poor
101. Shortness of breath
102. Shortened stride
103. Shoulders rounded forward

104. Sigh or yawn often
105. Singing long low tone sustains
106. Singing poorly
107. Snore
108. Soreness or pain in throat with "prolonged" vocal use
109. Sore deep pain feels like a band across your chest
110. Speech problems
111. Sports/exercise induced asthma
112. Stiff neck
113. Stressed out
114. Stomach tight-unable to let it go or you notice it letting   go, not having realized it was tense in the first place
115. Stroke
116. Sunken chest
117. Swallowing difficulty
118. Swim - can't at all, as well or as easily as you used to
120. Talking on the phone makes you short of breath
121. Tension around the eyes
122. Tense overall feeling (hypertension)
123. Thoughts run amuck
124. Tightness around mouth
125. Thoracic insufficiency syndrome
126. Tightness, soreness or pressure in the chest or

below   breast bone

127. Type "A"

128. Upper note singing problems

129. Upset stomach or irritable bowl syndrome

130. Vision blurred or eyesight better in AM than before   bed? Y__N__

131. Vocal or speech problems

132. Voice feels weak

133. Nervous quiver in voice

134. Wake from sleep suddenly not breathing = Apnea

135. Washboard abs

136. Wake up tired a lot

137. Wheezing

138. Mitral value prolapse

Write down the 3 items above you want MOST to improve:

_____

UDB© or **Unbalanced Dysfunctional Breathing** was first clarified by Michael G. White, Optimal Breathing® Coach. It's wise to eliminate UDB as it can severely hinder oxygenation and nervous system function. More about this at

http://www.breathing.com/articles/udb.htm and

http://www.breathing.com/articles/carbon-dioxide.htm

Optimal Breathing® Toll Free 866 MyInhale   **866 694 6425** *© 2004 Michael Grant White*

OPTIMAL BREATHING® PRIMARY EVALUATIONS HOW WELL YOU ARE BREATHING?

MAJOR FACTORS FOR HOW WELL YOU BREATHE – this is NOT a medical diagnostic. It is what we use to mark breathing development progress. See your physician if you think you might have a medical condition.

REGARDLESS OF THE DIAGNOSIS, IT IS OUR OPINION THAT IT WOULD BE VERY WISE TO DEVELOP YOUR BREATHING AT YOUR EARLIEST CONVENIENCE.

These evaluations are in a logical progressive order (not necessarily more important).

The previous **UDB** page is from both a subjective and objective perspective.

This approach is a deeper and more replicating and objective, focusing on simple and measurable change-ability. Improvement of these physical measurements will most often mean improvements in the UDB sheet.

1. List your UDB check sheet most significant issues

(in general and for this session).

What you pay more attention to and come back to - for gauging progress.

Fill out a new UDB page for each session. See the reductions/improvements or back slides.

---

2. What would you like to accomplish with your breathing development? _____

---

3. Blood Pressure: ____over____

4. Breath rate per minute _____

Resting Breath pauses: 2 sec; __1.5 sec; __ 1 sec; __.
5 sec;__ 0 sec;__ Tentative breath_____
(A *pause* is the length of time after the exhale, before you inhale.)
Follow your breathing and note in your mind the length of pauses between your complete breaths. (Use one thousand one, two thousand two, three thousand three, etc. to sense how long are your pauses.) Or have a friend keep time for you. Total_____

Less than 3 seconds?

A pause is the resting phase between the inhale and exhale. No pause, no rest. Some call this "a point of stillness." With too short a pause, your body never really rests. Using an automobile metaphor — your engine is still at high revolutions, even while at a stop sign. If your pauses are too short, you don't rest —even while sleeping!

Excessively long pauses (past 10 seconds) can be related to sleep disturbances, including sleep apnea, snoring and heart conditions.

Your breathing rate is the key; then comes the relationship between your breathing rate and pause. Pauses that are too short can cause chronic fatigue and stress.

Less than 3 seconds definitely requires change. No pause or less than a one second pause is a state of emergency and often accompanies severe maladies and negative conditions.

Shorter pauses generally relate to anxiety, panic attacks, heart conditions, high blood pressure and a general tendency to be less-than-healthy. (Highly recommend ordering our 176 video/DVD and Better Breathing Exercise #1).

5. Number count after two tries are the same_____.

This helps determine your breathing volume and oxygen uptake efficiency.

Lie, sit or stand. If you stand, then bend your knees slightly. Inhale as large as possible, then as quietly and quickly as possible, count and still be heard (*like a fast-whispering auctioneer*).Count to as high a number as you can on one full <u>exhale</u>. Write this number down and try it again. Try it a third time if you think the number will be much different.

(Note: during this exhalation number counting, do not:

    a. inhale b. skip any numbers c. hold your breath   d. breathe IN and count at the same time.)

If you reach 100 continue with one hundred one, one hundred two, and upward. Make sure you include the beginnings of each number, such as the "thirty" in thirty three , the "forty" in forty four, etc.

TEST REPEATS

Always repeat the tests again in whatever position (sitting, standing or lying) you did with the previous tests.

Ok, try it again.........

ANSWER

How high a number did you reach in that one long exhale? Total_____

Science has documented that your primary marker for longevity is the size (volume) of your breath. Your **Forced Exhalation Volume Oxygen** (FEV1) is primarily during the exhale. (Mike can reach 200-250!) How high a number count did you reach?

Try it again now if you are uncertain you did it properly.

My research strongly proves that counts below 100 indicate you most likely have a serious health challenge, or a condition that can invite one. Below 60? There is surely something wrong with your body, starting with your breathing. Please make absolutely sure that you take immediate action. Don't panic, don't worry, just take action and begin an **Optimal Breathing® Program** —soon!

6. Complete breaths — how many complete breaths per minute do you take? (at rest, while sitting or laying down —a complete breath = one inhale and one exhale plus varying lengths or any pause at the end of the exhale) Total _____

15 or more	**= Poor**
11-14	**= Fair**

8-10	= Good
5-7	= Very Good.
3-4	= Excellent

Higher breathing rates generally indicate a tendency towards, or actual state of, nervousness, anxiety, panic attacks, ranting and raving, heart conditions, high blood pressure, strokes, and a general state of less to far less than optimal breathing® and possible poor health. Poor breathing is a major cause of most health condition known to mankind.

To help reduce your breathing rate, order our *#176 DVD/video* and ***Better Breathing Exercise #1***. Focus on the program that seems most useable for your health condition. Your breath rate should reduce using our program. Just take the test above at least once a week to determine your progress.

http://www.breathing.com/programs.htm

7. Chest measurement

EXHALE____INHALE _____=_____

First take the TWO measurements.

a. Exhale as much as you can and take that measurement.

_____

b. Inhale as much as you can and take that measurement.

_____

c. Subtract the smaller one from the larger one and you have your chest expansion.

Record that number here_____.

Example:

Fully inhaled 37 1/4in.

Fully Exhaled = 35 in.

High chest expansion is 2.25 inches.

The more you try to increase the chest size and diaphragm strength by the effort of expelling the air, pursed lips exhale or blowing air exercises, wind instruments, and over exertion/breath heaving, the more the breathing system can become improved (somewhat), but still stiff, and lacking in expandability. The negative aspects are hardly noticed (if at all), because they occur in such small increments. If you have emphysema you will probably notice the difference immediately when the chest is expanded — even a little.

The rib, chest and shoulder muscles play as important a part in lung squeezing as the diaphragm. They passively support, or in many cases, can inhibit **Optimal Breathing®**. Movement and breathing are joined at the hip — pun intended! If you are not walking, moving, bending and breathing (such as with Yoga, Tai Chi, Feldenkrais, Alexander Technique, and Butoh), you should have someone helping you flex and stretch your rib cage. Pilates is especially helpful for geriatrics and people unable to move freely on their own. Dancers often breathe poorly due to their physical stresses, which are restrictive to their breathing. .

This measurement is also useful for measuring change every 3 months or so. During multi-session intensives, I often measure the client's chest expansion every day and have added up to a half inch in a single session. This expansion is most often maintained!

Between 1 & 2 inches is average. My educated guess is that if you are 5'2" and have one inch that is ok. Not good but ok. If you are 6'2" and have less than 2" that is not ok. A 5'2" singing client has a 3.5-inch expansion. For her size, this is excellent. Another client is 5'10" and had a 3/4-inch expansion. She is in big trouble. She also weighs 325 lbs.

(Mike's chest expansion is 4.5 inches. He is 6'2" and weighs 180 pounds.)

8. Do you raise your shoulders (at all) when taking a deep inhale? Y __ N ___

9. Do your neck muscles bulge out (at all) when you take a deep inhale? Y__ N ___

10. Observe and report your breathing quality (from UDB check sheet) _____

11. Voice quality: Strong even expressive voice._____ other_____

12. Squeeze and breathe_____ can you do it & feel it? Y ___ N ___

13. Respiratory faults? i.e. Ribs flare out or sunken chest or irregularly shaped rib cage?_____

14.Posture standing

relaxed_____rigid____collapsed_____forward flexion.

Y __ N __ palms facing inward ___ Knees stiff __ slightly bent_____ side leaning_____head tilted____

15. Chronic abdominal tension indicator: Breathe in: Does the belly go in __or out__. (Should go out.)

16. Voldynne score: (breathing volume inhalation tester) _____. (Not optimal volume measurement)

17. Capnometer (optional) more about at
http://www.breathing.com/articles/capnometry.htm

18. Breathing Scale:

A. Do you become severely out of breath when doing in heavy exercise? Date_____

B. Do you have to breathe harder than normal when walking on inclines or when you are hurrying on level ground? Date_____

C. Can you can still function adequately, but cannot keep up with people of your own age and physique during a stroll on level ground? Date_____

D. Does even the mildest exertion make you out of breath? Can you walk one city block or climb a flight of stairs without stopping to gasp for air? Date_____

Additional exercises for developing your Natural Breathing Reflex can be found on our
#176 DVD/video **and in the** *#191 Secrets manual.*

Chapter 4
Optimal Breathing® Results
Success Stories • Testimonials

There are hundreds more testimonials on our
http://www.breathing.com/results.htm pages.

Optimal Breathing® incorporates the best of all breathing development techniques and exercises. The people we work with come from a cross section of almost every job, race, religion, or lifestyle on Earth. **Optimal Breathing®** is generic for all humanity. The stories will give you a wide insight into the broad range of breathing development applications.

Our **Optimal Breathing®** system increases vital capacity, aspiratory capacity, functional reserve capacity, total lung capacity, tidal volume, and expiratory reserve volume. It decreases lung dead spaces and non- functional alveoli. It also invites increased oxygen uptake/utilization (QO_2) and reduced oxygen cost of breathing. Breathing patterns and breathing coordination are improved in all cases.

Improved breathing shows immediate benefits in these areas:
☆ **Stress and Tension, Coping and Relaxation**
☆ **Self-Improvement and Personal Growth**
☆ **Acute and Chronic Pain Management**

- ☆ **Emotional Disturbances and Behavioral Problems**
- ☆ **Substance Abuse and Recovery**
- ☆ **Creative and Athletic Performance**
- ☆ **Meditation and Martial Arts**
- ☆ **General Health and Well Being**
- ☆ **Life Extension and Longevity**
- ☆ **Psychic Skills and Intuitive Development**
- ☆ **Group Dynamics and Interpersonal Relations**
- ☆ **Spiritual Purification and Enlightenment**

Overview

According to Andrew Weil, M.D., Clinical Professor of Internal Medicine, University of Arizona in Tucson, "The simplest and most important technique for protecting your health is breathing. I have seen breath control alone achieve remarkable results: lowering blood pressure, ending heart arrhythmia, improving long-standing patterns of poor digestion, increasing blood circulation throughout the body, decreasing anxiety and allowing people to get off addictive anti-anxiety drugs and improving sleep and energy cycles."

"Like many people, I thought breathing was just something we did naturally....until I took some voice lessons, and learned a little about breathing correctly. Your site is teaching me even more."
Ann

A champion swimmer wanted to improve her ease of breathing and recovery times for multiple general race days and championship triathlete events. An opera singer was losing her high notes and sought psychotherapy but eventually just learned to breathe better and her high notes returned. A classical singer was losing her mid-range and regained it with Optimal Breathing® techniques. An emphysema victim learned that breathing was not what he thought is was for over 50 years. It had become a permanent misunderstanding even to the point of doing it improperly when shown the proper way. Sixteen sessions were needed to change this person's breathing. An asthmatic was retrained to breathe easier and the symptoms disappeared. Stuttering and spasmodic dysphonia can reduce or disappear when one learns to breathe optimally. A shy young lady learned to breathe better. Her shyness reduced and "I met a man and got married". Some eliminated their sleep problems, hypertension, type "A" responses, wimpy ways of being. Some increased their energy many fold, told off their suppressive boss, told the truth to their spouse, opened up to loving themselves, and set boundaries where needed. Some healed from illness or near death. There are thousands of stories like theseÉ!

Asthma

Learning to breathe under the guidance of Mike White has not only saved my life but profoundly altered its quality.

The first training session, Mike addressed my restricted breathing, which was steadily becoming worse, despite the inhalers I was using three and four times a day. He taught me the Leg Lift and shhhh breath, a deceptively simple and powerfully effective breath which stopped (within days) my chronic coughing, and began to clear and relieve lungs and bronchial tubes desperate for air.

Mike also used carefully controlled hand pressure and other techniques to "wring out and soften hard and atrophied lung tissue. This "re-birthing" of my lungs has affected my entire being. The relief from asthma turned out to be only an introduction into fuller and more vibrant participation in life. In the process of learning to breathe more deeply and easily, old fears and insecurities are beginning to dissolve. I am discovering the joyful calm that supports life at its base.

I believe Michael Grant White's work with the breath is a critically important contribution to an area of scientific research still in its infancy. An M.D. in California.

CHEST PAINS, shortness of breath, high blood pressure

I tried emailing this testimonial sometime in May but it never got through. Since then my daughters have been urging me to send in my testimonial because of how much your breathing exercises have helped me "cure" my chest pains, shortness of breath and lower my blood pressure. So I am sending it in now hoping this does get through to you.

I need to thank God for leading me to your website back in March when I began experiencing mild to severe chest pains every night. I had gone through a full bottle of 30 nitroglycerine tablets within two weeks. My chest pains always occurred at night when I am going to bed, so much so, that I was afraid to go to bed. I need to explain something, Mike. Because of my past two open heart surgeries and heart problems, I am quite knowledgeable about the symptoms of a possible heart attack when you experience chest pains. In my case, I had just gone through an ultra sonic and a treadmill test in February. During the treadmill test, at the final stage, I complained to the attending nurse that she had to stop the treadmill because I was experiencing severe chest pains and was out

71

of breath. She insisted I continue because the test was almost over and I needed to go on just for another minute or so. Somehow I got through the run and nearly fainted, heaving and breathing rapidly.

Two weeks later when I returned to my cardiologist for the results of my test, the cardiologist stated that I had over 75% blockage on my right carotid artery and 50% blockage on my left carotid artery. He immediately recommended an angiogram to determine the actual extent of the blockage. After consulting with my wife, I decided to forego the angiogram and in fact vowed that I would not go through that invasive examination again. Right after that was when I started to experience my chest pains. However, as I mentioned to my wife, the chest pains that I was experiencing could not be heart related but instead, I suspected it may be initiating from my lungs. After my treadmill test, I also started to cough out some mucous. Its color was pure white and not yellow or black so I felt that I may have a latent lung problem.

After all, I am over 73 tears old. Besides during my chest pains, I did not experience any of the usual symptoms of a pending heart attack. I felt like I couldn't breathe and the center of my chest hurt badly. The pain vanished after I slipped a nitro tablet under my tongue. My blood pressure was not low at the time but it wasn't high either. Of course I was frightened. I would get chest pains for two or three nights, then none on the next night, and then it started again. About that time, I read an article in our local newspaper about breathing. I went on the internet and I can't tell you how or why I selected your web site. I spent all day reading the information on your site especially the testimonials. I ordered your Optimal Breathing package and received the tapes in early April.

Now, let me tell you what happened!

I started out on the middle of my living room floor, arranging some couch pillows on a towel on the floor. Didn't take me long to adjust myself on the floor and started with the Tibetan Caffeine tape. As God is my witness, by the time I was into the second half of the tape and into the exhale and inhale on a single bong strike, my right leg from my thigh to my feet felt like ice. I continued my breathing exercises and had my wife cover my legs with a blanket. I went through the entire exercise which took me nearly an hour that very first time. Mike, that night I did not have any chest pain. I did the same exercise twice the next day, once in the morning and then again before going to bed.

The second night, my chest pain returned, but this time instead of taking a nitro tablet, I went into the living room and sat on the edge of my couch and in the dark, started to breath slowly. The chest pain slowly subsided and after a few minutes it was gone and I was able to go to bed. From that day on I have had no chest pains and have not taken a nitro tablet. This all happened in April after I started with your breathing exercises.

Today, I do breathing almost the entire day, mostly subconsciously be causing the breathing exercises are part of my daily routine. There is a lot more I can tell you about my health as a result of the breathing exercises I learned from you. My daughter who lives in Hawaii has just visited you in North Carolina and I am grateful for the teaching and help you have given her. I have told my youngest daughter about the Tibetan Caffeine (Better Breathing Exercise 2) and she too will be doing the healing breathing exercises herself. In closing here is my email address, *bobby7778@hotmail.com* for anyone who is fortunate enough to find your website, they can contact me and I would be happy to tell

them how wonderful breathing the right way can be for them
Aloha   — Bruno Yim

CHEST PAINS

Aloha Mike! I am ordering your tapes because my Dad has had great improvement in his health with them (testimonial above). He was having chest pains (after two bypass surgeries) and high blood pressure, both of which subsided/went down, after practicing the Better Breathing Exercises #2 for a month. He is 73yrs. and sounded very pleased and enthusiastic - the best I've heard him in years!

M.I.T Trained Biochemist

Of all the essential nutrients needed by the human, oxygen is the one we must have on a moment to moment basis; we can't live without it even for a few minutes. Yet this is the one nutrient most people don't associate with deficiency problems. Nothing could be further from the truth.. One problem is that oxygen concentrations in and around major cities have been measured as much as 30% below normal. That means that each breath brings in less oxygen. As if this weren't bad enough, most people have developed poor breathing habits, thus further restricting oxygen intake. The resulting oxygen deficiency is having a negative effect on our health and our overall performance.

Oxygen deprivation can be associated with all kinds of chronic diseases, including cancer. Michael White is an extraordinary breathing coach who teaches people new patterns of breathing, helping them to bring in more oxygen. These techniques help to improve health, stamina and even voice quality. — Raymond Francis, Director, Beyond Health Corporation

Raw-Living Foods Chef Phillip Madeley

I highly recommend the work of Michael Grant White. It has touched my life on a very profound level. Excellent breathing is absolutely essential to everything in our lives. It provides energy, assists digestion, improves brain efficiency and assists in providing optimal body functioning. Breathing for me though is much more. Breathing correctly has allowed me to tap into the magical side of life... the spirit within!

Through learning how to breathe in the whole body we can go beyond the mind and our animalistic thinking. Most of us breathe in the chest area stimulating the sympathetic (Flight or Fight) nervous system. This incorrect breathing began at birth with our conditioning, civilized life's non stop emotional upheaval, polluted cites and increased stress without the release.

By learning how to breathe we can bring our breath down and learn to stay in the parasympathetic (slowing down, restorative) nervous system for most of the time. In times of crisis we can use optimal breathing development and exercises to bring it back there.

The practice of Mike's exercises allows the natural reflexive breathing to be rehabilitated.

Basically we are retraining our body to breathe naturally, so these are not just short term exercises, they are designed to recondition and reorganize the way we breathe.

One of my favorite exercises was not a specific breath exercise, but a Qi Gong exercise. This simple exercise, taught in his Secrets of Optimal Breathing manual, of standing still in relaxed posture has revolutionized my own posture and thus increased my breathing capacity. The Better Breathing Exercise #2 (aka Tibetan Caffeine), singing exercises, the shhh breath have also opened up my breath and lungs like never before. Two years later I still practice the techniques and exercises because I get results from them. While working with Mike in 2000 I was introduced to a strapping exercise which really allows an opening and expanding of lung capacity, Mike has a video that you can use at home for this.

The changes for me were very subtle, yet like any true natural health practice, accumulative over time. And I have not even practiced them daily!!

So don't despair if you don't get immediate results, though many do. Just persevere and gradually your breathing will open on a whole new level.

Excellent breathing in conjunction with living foods, yoga and meditation, provides you with the tools that may enable you to find your peace... whatever life throws at you. Phillip Madeley http://www.sattvic-life.com http://www.freshupnorth.com http://www.breathing.com/energy-5-level.htm Level 3

Chiropractor

Mike White is truly a master of the breath. As a long time martial artist, chiropractor and singer, I thought I had a handle on breathing. What I created was non-optimal breathing patterns by over emphasizing the abdominal aspect of the breath. This was depriving me of the fullest expansion possible. Mike's due diligence and keen powers of observation helped me open up. As I breathe easier I am letting go of patterns of effort in my life. The breath is truly a living metaphor. Thank you, Mike! — David Miller, D.C.

From Gay Hendricks

If you've never seen Mike's powerful work, you're in for a real transformational treat. You'll see why he's simply called The Breathing Coach. You can check out his work at www.breathing.com.

Migraines, chest pains, vitality and emotions

Just wanted to tell you how much I enjoy your newsletter. My sister ------ was fortunate to have had the opportunity to meet with you in early June. She mentioned what a kind person you are. She lives in Hawaii, I in Nevada, but we talk with each other several times a week and she has continued working with her breathing. On her way back from North Carolina, she stopped in Nevada to join us in celebrating my daughter's high school graduation, and shared with us what she has learned.

I have had terrible migraines for several years now and just this week, I tried some of your techniques for breathing (properly!) and lo and behold, they first subsided and then eventually disappeared. How wonderful it was to rid myself of this. I will continue these techniques whenever I feel the need. In closing, please keep me informed if you plan on visiting Las Vegas.

My father who also lives in Las Vegas, uses your tapes, etc. as faithfully as my sister and I know he would love to join me in going to any seminars/classes that you may present. He was experiencing chest pains (angina?) periodically and since he started his **Optimal Breathing® Program**, he has not touched his nitroglycerine. It is amazing given his history of heart disease. He also feels more vital. The greatest reward is that even emotionally, he has opened himself up to us all. I thank you, Mike, as there are many more things that have happened to our family since meeting you. Sincerely, D. M.

Weight Loss

I learned to breathe better and right from the start I had more energy and felt more like exercising.

— Katherine H. Computer programmer

Retired Athletics Instructor

You took professional interest in my health situation, and have given me so much helpful information. I am forever grateful! For over 50 years, I taught aerobics, water exercise, swimming, dancing, and helped people to relax to reduce their pain. Your breathing information is a help in ALL of these activities and situations as well as improving health and enjoyment of life. MT, retired.

Anxiety

I was looking at the animated lungs on your website home page. I started imitating what I was observing on the screen. Man, did I notice a difference or what!!!!!!!!

I can't believe the difference it's making on my levels of anxiety. I feel a lot better. I feel convinced that I can bring about (as is pointed out in the cybercast) a significant improvement in my frame of mind.

I know it's only a minor effort in comparison to what I can get from studying the kit or attending a workshop (which I intend to do), but, I am now committed to learning to breathe, whereas before I only understood it on an intellectual level.. Now I KNOW it works.

I'm finding ways to get the word out to as many people as possible... sending your site address to some friends. Thanks for getting the message out. You're the Man!   Pat Walsh

Orthopedic Specialist

I thoroughly enjoyed my session with you. I was delighted by the degree of insight and sophistication that you bring to "breathing". I am now opening up and breathing in a much more relaxed manner. I look forward to another session to go a step further. I will also be recommending your approach to my patients. – Dr. Richard Gracer, Orthopedic Medicine

Internist

Our modern medical paradigm bases pulmonary function on factors that relate to the anatomy and physiology of the lungs. At times, the mechanical relationships of the chest cavity and of the diaphragm are considered important, but for the most part, they are rarely considered in the ordinary management of most pulmonary diseases such as emphysema, asthma, and restrictive lung disorders.

The bulk of our management of these kinds of disorders is aimed at pharmacological intervention. While this is a reasonable approach that often is quite valuable, it fails to appreciate the potential role of posture, rib flexibility or diaphragmatic excursion as independent factors that can improve lung function. This can be life saving to people with severe pulmonary insufficiency.

It would be unheard of in the development of opera singing, powerful public speaking, or world class athletics to ignore the importance of respiratory faults, accessory breathing muscles, and breathing coordination. When the pulmonary reserves of these highly trained specialists are examined, they are clearly superior to that of the average, untrained population. There have been but few clinical studies undertaken to explore the seemingly obvious benefits of this kind of training..

It seems prudent to me to explore this safe, non-invasive, and easily taught approach, to patients who are willing to invest a minimum of money and time especially when the potential for a negative effect with selected exercises is zero. When conventional therapies have little or nothing to offer, searching for additional possibilities becomes our responsibility. — Len Saputo, MD

Asthmatic

I'm cutting back on the use of my inhaler..– Mark D.

Brahma Bull Rider

My vertigo is gone after 10 years of unsteady walking. Rich. C., Brahma Bull Rider

Chi Kung

I wanted to tell you how effective I found your techniques for improving breath capacity and a sense of smoothing out the mechanics of both my inhale and exhale. I drew the best breath of my life after you used the "strapping" method.

I also appreciate your efforts with the football players, and your work with the strength and conditioning coach that so remarkably improved their performance in the timed drills. The return to fluid movement, even after they had been pushed to exhaustion, showed how effective your techniques were in their improved performance and comfort under duress. — J. Michael Wood, Chairman of The Board (2004) NQA, National Qigong Association

Therapeutic Bodyworker

Mike has the skill, the depth of experience and the commitment to guide you beyond yourself to new horizons of capacity. — Gary Hagman, Therapeutic Bodyworker

Chronic Pain

My pain is manageable without medication. I sleep better too. LT, Retired

Psychotherapist

Working with you I'm able to access feelings stored in my body that I can't access with words.
– Joan P. MFCC, Psychotherapist

Better Sleep

I can sleep all night for the first time in 20 years. — Rose W., retired

Stuttering

After forty years of stuttering I'm now stuttering much less. – Mary W

EMPHYSEMA

Learn every day by reading your posts. I realize how lucky I am when I read of the problems of others. Twenty years ago I started going downhill in what was called lung capacity. First they told me I was 30% then twenty---and recently they just checked to see if I need oxygen. They quote a figure of under 15 but say the figures mean little as some who are 20% capacity can equal those who are 40%..

The interesting thing I have for you all is the past year I HAVE IMPROVED!!!! I owe it all to the internet and a person named Mike White whom I never met. He is called The Breathing Coach and you can learn how to help yourself by reading his website. I can't wait for an appointment if he is ever in my area. Everything is cheap compared to hospitals, medicines and not breathing well.

The site is free and he will give you help free. I doubled my walking capacity within three months by reading his website and devoting an hour a day to his advice. After that I bought one of his inexpensive books and progressed more. I am excited. Look it over-- two Doctors have told me ---can't hurt. check After a week you will say "There is something to it" Don ---Fl.

Sleep Apnea

My sleep apnea is gone after twenty five years and my asthma is lessening. – Mark B.

High Blood Pressure

After five years of using prescription drugs to unsuccessfully control my high blood pressure, your breathing exercise finally got the job done. I feel great! – Judith P., Interior Designer

Triathlete

After the last session with you my running really smoothed out and my recovery time is much lower.   – Jeff S., Triathlon contestant.

Workshop Attendee

You mean all I have to do to feel this good is to breathe? – Joan R..

Phobic Trial Attorney

I just crossed the San Rafael bridge doing your breathing exercise and my fear of crossing bridges is gone. – Kelly K., Trial Attorney

Pranayama Student

I just wanted to express my appreciation for your web-site and, what I suspect is your passion. My experience with pranayama and other eastern breath practices for going on 25 years has been, shall we say, a "learning" experience. The path I took would have been better served having had someone like yourself around to correct the unintended mistakes (learning from experience is not always the best way). My current understanding certainly supports and agrees with your well-written perceptions. Thank you. Gary A, NC

Chronic Obstructive Pulmonary Disease (COPD)

Thank you for sending the "Secrets of Optimal Natural Breathing" to me so promptly. I did get it in plenty of time to take it to .... with me. There I simply read it several times without trying to do any exercises or assessments.

In the past few days I have been trying to work with the exercises. I have also worked with the tape once. I intend to continue all this because already I have had some significant help.

I do plan to come up for some individual work in the next few months. I am quite taken by your work. I recently finished a pulmonary rehab program at Vanderbilt University; and this morning when I walked (hobbled for a few blocks) I thought: "Well everything I did in that program was a kind of forcing; and now for the first time, I am glimpsing what it means to take a real breath."

When I got home my oxygen saturation jumped up to 99% for the first time. Thanks a lot. I have a long way to go. In addition to my COPD I am now struggling to recover from a back injury. I will continue with your basic exercises for awhile and let you know when I might make a trip. — Thanks, Phyllis P

SPEAKING

You can read as many books as you like, watch as many videos or read as many web sights as you can. It is the Realized knowledge that hits you in the back of the head when you least expect it that grabs you and changes your consciousness and understanding of any subject. As you know I have taken an interest in your breathing exercises (probably doing them wrong, but I'm doing them). I especially like the Tibetan Caffeine exercises. Any way, I was at work yesterday. I work for a large recently merged corporation where there is a dismal aspect of life due to many rifs (reduction in force layoffs). Lots of shallow breathing there! Not to mention lots of over-perfumed people to wreak havoc with those of us who have sensitivity to such airborne "solvents". One of my colleagues became extremely sick -sneezing and coughing wheezing etc. I could feel my own lungs tightening up too.

I went outside in the fresh air and did a series of your caffeine breaths (had to imagine the bowl strikes) 15 minutes later, I came back in to the office and started talking in what I thought would be my normal voice and out came the voice of a stronger –healthier and much "larger" man! –or so it seemed. I was truly amazed at the difference in my voice after this brief exercise session.

I was not sure that I could see the link between your questions about voice quality on your free breathing test but I do now. It is interesting to me to have rather inadvertently observed this correlation between quality, depth, rhythm of breath and voice sound.. M.A., Boston Mass

Manic Depression

My breathing feels locked up and when I unlock it, I go from anxious and angry to calm and relaxed. Walt P. (This man has steel rods on each side of his spine in about 8 vertebrae because of an accident that almost killed him. These rods freeze up his natural reflexes and take his nervous system out of balance).

Manic Depression-bipolar

I've been so much more stable for months now that I am starting to work with my doctor to back away from my medication. Nick D.

Relieving the Trauma of Mammography

As a believer in natural healing, I have managed to stay away from allopathic medicine for the last 30 years. My main reason for stepping into the medical world again was to get a prescription for natural (bioidentical) hormones. To rule out tumors, I was required to have a mammogram (my first). As hard as the clinic tried to make this a pleasant experience (15 minute massage, lovely surroundings, caring staff), I felt thoroughly traumatized and came home exhausted.

For the 6 days following the mammogram, I experienced a lot of soreness beneath each breast. My side ribs were also very sore and hurt when I inhaled. What was more distressing was my emotional and mental state. I had just received my breathing kit from Michael Grant White and I called him to see which one of his breathing

85

techniques would move me out of distress the fastest. He instructed me in a special technique using a strap included with the 176 video.

I tried it two or three times and noticed a lessening of pain and distress each time. Feeling encouraged, I used the technique 2 or 3 more times. After 30 minutes or so, the physical pain was 95% gone and what is even more significant, my emotional and mental distress was gone. In its place was a feeling of calm and much more room in my chest to breathe. I continued to do more of the *Better Breathing Exercise #2* and was pleasantly surprised to find a substantial improvement in my breathing after doing the exercise only one time. — C.P., San Diego,CA

From Mike: *Massage therapists will tell you that pain from mammograms is quite common. There may be many women that can benefit from the above technique Carol refers to. As always check with your doctor first.*

Breathing, Trauma, Tightness In Chest & Personal Power
Breath Coaching Sessions with Michael Grant White
by Alan Paul

I was a long term severely abused child, physically and emotionally. I am steadfastly determined to improve my sense of wholeness, to strengthen my self-esteem and self-love and spiritual connection with others. As a result of this commitment, I have spent much of the last 30 years looking for help with my breathing, which has always (since adolescence) felt tense and shallow and "locked up" and eventually led to me having to give up my chosen profession.

Over the years, I've tried every type of healing modality I could think of that might impact the experience of never being able to get a satisfying breath. I've tried medical doctors, chiropractic, various psychotherapies including Psychoanalytic, Gestalt, Short-Term Psychodynamic, and others. I've tried body-oriented therapies including Reichian, Alexander Technique, Rebirthing, Rolfing, Rosen Work, Biofeedback, Massage Therapy, Bioenergetics, Core Energetics, Primal, Reiki, Cranio-Sacral, etc.. I also studied Yoga and Tai Chi. For many of these modalities I tried more than one practitioner of that style. I also committed extensive periods of time to a number of these practitioners, many of whom I studied with for periods of 1 to 3 years, in hope of getting some help.

While some of these teachers and therapists were very smart and dedicated people who were able to help me move forward in one way or another, no one was able to help me find relief from my core complaint my inability to breathe satisfactorily.

Eventually, I decided to travel to North Carolina for a week, to work intensively with Mike. He started by showing me how some simple adjustments to my posture could give me more space to breathe, eliminating tightness in my chest. He then, using very specific rib/chest/shoulder/neck accessory breathing muscle release techniques went on to show me how to get the ribs and diaphragm moving so that the breath could expand into the increased space he had found for me in my posture. Some of the beliefs that I had held about what a coordinated breathing feels like, had to be corrected.

Finally, there was a wonderful moment with Mike when everything "clicked" for me, and I was able to sing loudly and happily with no pain or straining, for the first time I can remember since early childhood. Mike was able to get me back to the same state again, and I eventually returned home with a set of exercises and "homework" to do to help continue the development. I was quite satisfied and happy with my lessons with Mike.

But the biggest changes became apparent when I returned home. Suddenly, conversations with associates had a different character, the movement of my ribs seemed huge compared to before I traveled to North Carolina. A close associate has commented that I seem noticeably more relaxed. My dreams are much more vivid (some pleasant, some not so pleasant). A low-grade depression seems to have lifted, and I suddenly find myself easily working long hours whereas that was difficult for months before my trip.

I've also noticed an odd and unexpected difference in my diet after years of complacency, I've begun eating salads every day and generally eating less overall. Food is still very enjoyable, but it seems less like entertainment and comfort to me, and more like...well...food. Somehow, breathing a little deeper and easier has, without any conscious effort to do so, made me more realistic and less emotionally clouded about diet.

Another thing that changed immediately after returning home, is my exercise routines. I generally swim every day and do a good bit of flexibility work every day. But after studying with Mike, I'm beginning to feel that there really is only one form of exercise breathing development. Everything else (swimming, stretching, weight-training, tai chi, running, you name it) is just a variation of breathing development.

For example, when I swim now, I'm very conscious of moving my limbs and ribs in such a way that the breath deepens with every stroke, so that the breath is more expansive and elastic when I get out of the pool than when I got in. This is quite different than the way I used to swim. I swam a lot harder than I swim now, and there was a general sense of triumph and temporary relaxation in that, but the relaxation didn't extend to my breath, which was tight and shallow when I was finished. Mike has assured me that I'll swim even stronger than before, if I'm careful to slowly increase the cardio demand such that the breathing apparatus remains relaxed. I always thought that the more cardio fitness, the better, as long as one doesn't have a heart attack.

But I've learned that you can do quite a bit of subtle damage to the enjoyment of your life (and even your long-term health) by placing athletic demands on your body that are out of synch with your breathing abilities. So breathing comes first for me now, particularly since Mike's given me some tools with which to increase my breath.

I've noticed the same thing with my stretch routines. I no longer believe that there's such a thing as an "ankle stretch." Sure, I do the same ankle routines as before, but the way I do them is completely different. So there's no ankle stretches. Just "breath stretches" extended out to the ankles.

Mike also talked to me repeatedly about the ergonomics of my life in my easy chair, my work chair , my car seat. When Mike discussed these things, I listened and thought he made some good points worth considering. But since I've returned home, I'm beginning to feel that he was talking about something really important_. I can see how slouching at my desk for a couple of hours leaves me with less breath, and that then induces a feeling of low self-esteem and depression. I guess I never noticed before because I didn't feel that I had all that much breath to protect. Now, with my breath deeper, I'm beginning to think seriously about how to improve my ergonomics (Mike gave me a number of good and inexpensive suggestions.)

Just now, as I sat and wrote this, I realized that I am indeed slouching and locking up my breath. I need to replace this desk chair with a more breathing-friendly chair (not a specialty item, just an inexpensive but different chair design than I'm currently using), in accordance with the suggestions that Mike gave me. So I got up and did about 10 minutes of my breathing exercises. Now, sitting back down to work, it's easier to work, the words are flowing with less effort, my self-esteem is higher, I feel more confident, life seems less like a burden. It's subtle, but tangible. No, it's not magic, my life isn't suddenly euphoric. But it's easier, less work, more filled with hope and promise, than it was 10 minutes ago. It makes me wonder how many of my internal conflicts and frustrations are nothing more than the effects of poor breathing habits.

Some people tell me let go of the past, grieve the losses, forgive those who hurt you, move on toward life. They mean well by encouraging me to fly, but they assume that I have the wings with which to fly. How can I grieve the past and move on, if my breathing is locked up so that I can't fully laugh, cry, or sing?

Mike has helped me see some of the possibilities for correcting my breathing pattern, and the results of that have been simple and immediate. It feels good to breathe better. And it's very reassuring to know that there are specific exercises I can do for my breath, that will help me to let go of the past and create the future. AP.

Shortness of breath, dyslexia

After years of living short of breath I made a choice to get from

Orlando to North Carolina to visit Michael White to see if he could correct my ways of breathing.

On arrival I wanted to get straight in to the learning experience, telling Michael that my biggest concern is the escape of air when talking and the breathiness that has created unnecessary tension that I could and need to live with out. The tension that has created over the last few years is causing me to hold my breath. This causes not living life to the fullest as my mind seems to wander instead of focusing on what is going on in present time.

After discussing the importance of "breath" which I was greatly aware of due to my own ongoing training in exercises and activities such as, Yoga, balanced diet and meditation.

Throughout my two days visit we did a range of hands-on techniques and exercises,

After going over many details, I realized that the in breath is something that requires no self-conscious effort at all, but to unlearn the thoughtful "conscious" breath is a hard long way to conquer, but very much worth it.

Michael showed a way to a very relaxing ease of talking with a lot of tension release. To my surprise I felt that my body was at one, head connected to my rest of my body, it gives you internal strength.

Another exercise was a gentle, but firm press on my neck, relieving tension I noticed in an instance, eyes seemed to be more relaxed and my head felt that it was on correctly on my shoulder.

The counting numbers exercises was a baseline and marking progress exercise to see how fast air escapes. My first count was 20. Which is something I had to work on. After a while worked my way up to the 50, then 65.

Having been told of my Dyslexia over the past years I was

accustomed to it and placed this in the back of my brain. When Michael asked me to say out loud the alphabet I mentioned that I was never able to speak it out correctly, partly due my Dyslexia. Within 10 minutes I was saying it out loud, accurately repeated and for the rest of my life. Perhaps I gave up on it a long time a go, it is a big mental plus.

One exercise showed me how much I was off the average target of rib expansion, comparing mine with Michael's; it was about a 200% difference in Michael's favor. That is my target.

All in all, it was very interesting visit; with a lot of information to take home, it was not a quick fix as I hoped for. But the information given to me makes me able to set my self-free, it is up to me and I have the right tools to get there. I've seen what can be done and what needs to be done. — Steven. Harberts

From a Licensed Massage Therapist:

I am an Licensed Massage Therapist in Florida. All through school and since I have been searching for something to specialize in that will make a difference to those I touch.

My wife, also and LMT, was speaking to a peer about the seminars that she took and which one of them most benefited her, she replied "OPTIMAL BREATHING" by Mike White. So my wife and I looked up the website and researched the whole site. As I read through the many links and pages, I knew I was onto something. I called Mike and arranged for my wife and I to take the intensive course. I thought this course would bring more of a balanced circle of my breathing techniques since I have already learned the Yoga Breath and many other techniques of breathing.

What fascinated me most about Mike's work was the

MECHANICAL part of my breathing. How can anyone improve breathing by any other means UNLESS one can begin by breathing correctly to BEGIN WITH. To re-set the internal mechanism and breathe correctly, to set a new foundation to breathing is the ONLY way to get more out of other types of breathing. Also, to add this technique to my practice appeared beneficial. It occurred to me that this component of health care was (and still is) missing. Remember the days when you went to the doctor and they examined you in a gown, with nothing on underneath it? They checked everything, eyes, ears, nose, throat, heart rate and even that cold stethoscope up against your chest and actually listened to you breath!

Those days are gone, and the medical world is missing the boat big time on not checking the respirations of their patients. BREATH IS LIFE...Correct breathing is living that life more fully, enthusiastically, vitally with mobility and longevity. Mike's course gives you that and much more. Taking fuller, richer, deeper breaths with pauses in between the exhale and inhale most definitely provides more energy, stamina and ATP (Adenosine Triphosphate) for the body to function more peacefully with less effort. Since returning home, I have incorporated these techniques into my daily living with positive results. I am making vital decisions in my business more quickly and efficiently.

No more irritability (my wife likes that part) I have sustained energy, even with 12-14 hour days. I just plain KNOW that I am healthier. Also, I am integrating these techniques into my practice with clients and getting very positive results. Anyone wondering if they should or should not invest the time and money into this program only need ask themselves one question "To BREATHE or not to BREATHE?"

This course is worth every dime and then some. I will be taking the advanced courses and absorb more information to further my quest to genuinely make a difference in the health care system as I withdraw from the "SICK CARE" system currently in place. — Dennis L. Bradley, LMT Jacksonville, FL

Choir Leader

I've been a singing professional for years but you showed me a new way. My power, singing ease and flexibility increased incredibly and I handle levels of voice, fear and energy that would have crushed me just a short while ago. – Linda Webb Kakaba., Published and Touring Singer/Songwriter

Breath is life, but for the flautist breath is also art. Working with Mike freed tensions that had built up through years of playing so I was able to recover my full capacity, control and ease of expression. I recommend him highly top anyone who wants to maximize his or her breathing capability. — Leslie Newman, Member Toronto Symphony 2003

Classical Singer

My high notes have returned to stay. – Maria H., Opera singer preparing for Carnegie Hall performance

Seminar Leader

Thanks for helping to improve my breathing. As a result, my seminars on selling homes to people from diverse culture have much more power and impact."– Michael Lee.

Stage Fright

It's gone. Just gone. — Jim Brown. Trumpet player

Stuttering

After forty years of stuttering I'm now stuttering much less. – Mary W

Fear of Speaking in Public

It's gone. For the first time ever, it's GONE. Thank God. — Ben Warren

Singing

Yes I wish to subscribe to your newsletter. As a singer, good breathing is simply a necessity. A good technique frequently becomes confused by "so called" knowledgeable teachers. Your site is great. Thank you for all the info you share. It is sure to be helpful to many. Judy Davis.

TESTIMONIALS & IMPORTANT INSIGHTS FROM OPTIMAL BREATHING® SCHOOL GRADUATES & APPRENTICES

I am finding watching the almost immediate results so rewarding and the expressions on the children's faces as they realize the ease in breathing and the difference it makes them feel is incredible. Thank you for it all and hope all is well — Karen Walker, Private Tutor, Sidney Australia

MEDICAL QIGONG MASTER

First I would like to thank you for the training to become an Optimal Breathing Development Specialist Apprentice (OBDSA). Not only was the "hands on" training a great learning experience, but it helped me get the "feel" required to work with patients and clients.

An added benefit was discovering the glitches in my own breathing mechanics and posture, and the chance to use the Optimal Breathing techniques to correct them during our classes. It was particularly notable that I was able to reduce my pulse rate by 6 beats/min., and increase my blood oxygen level by 3% in just 5-6 breaths after correcting the problem. I have now been able to create the "over the top" breathing experience at will, and the paradox of more relaxation and more energy is constantly present.

I also noticed that while I was doing Qigong meditation in the supine position and using the Primary Rest Position, I had one of the best energetic meditations I have experienced in 4 years! I will be looking forward to the results I achieve in moving meditation.

The backrest you made for my automobile allowed me to make the 4 1/2 hour drive home after the workshop without feeling the fatigue I normally experience. I was able to draw deep, relaxed breaths while driving with the backrest and the seat angle changes you recommended. I thank you, and my back thanks you!

Thank you again for sharing your knowledge, experience and enthusiasm in our class. It will provide a lifetime of relief for me, and I will be able to pass it along to the people I will work with in my practice.

— J. Michael Wood, PBMC, OBDSA ,Medical QiGong Mastert. Nashville, TN

A young man on a spiritual path

When I signed up to spend four days with Mike White, I expected to learn a lot about how to deal with other people's breathing problems. What I didn't expect was to have a life changing experience that continues to affect me on a daily basis.

I had never really made the connection between breathing and your voice. But by using singing and breathing exercises I was able to clear and strengthen my voice. And what a difference it makes! My confidence grew a huge amount, and in such a short amount of time it was astonishing.

That was one of the most important lessons I gained from Mike: that progress doesn't have to take years. In fact, huge progress can be made in a matter of minutes!

Another area that exceeded my expectations was that of overall health. Mike was not just interested in my breathing alone, but my whole entire body. I learned dietary changes, and exercise routines that would help my body to stay healthy and breathing optimally.

And of course my breathing was the thing that improved the most. I did gain a good amount of lung capacity, but what was even more important to me was the rhythm of my breathing. Before, I had a very fast, very shallow breath. Through many different exercises, including strap work, body work, voice work and coaching, I was able to dramatically slow my breath down, and deepen my natural breath. This deepening of the automatic breath still brings me wonder as every breath I take, without any effort on my part, feels slow and deep.

The effect of these changes has included deeper sleeping, more energy, and most importantly a raising of my level of consciousness. Things are much clearer than they were before, and my health has taken an even higher priority in my life. The importance of breathing has finally taken its proper place. Thanks Mike! — Aaron Butler, Sedona Az.

From Leiah Carr, LMT,RM,CH

I attended the Optimal Breathing course at ....I was very excited abut the class, even before it occurred, as I had learned about, and experienced the Optimal Breathing techniques through a fellow therapist. Rebecca Sharp had taken the course and had carried a great deal of enthusiasm about the work, and the impact it has on health.

Having personally experienced some of the therapy, I was very eager to learn the method for myself. My practice is in Jacksonville, The (name withheld pending level 2 outcome) has a primary focus of working with individuals to educate and provide methods to achieve and maintain optimum health. The Optimal Breathing techniques seemed like another wonderful tool to add ton the many varied things I already use, depending on the individual needs of each client. In the class it was emphasized what you can not have optimum health without proper breathing.

To experience the strapping techniques by several different practitioners during the course was also a great experience. Each practitioner had their own uniqueness that added depth to the program. Each practitioner shared their feedback and questions that helped make the experience broader and richer for me.

The techniques that were learned were simple and straightforward, but powerful in their effects. The understanding of the importance of the diaphragm, and the body's need for a full healthy breath was very enlightening. to learn the techniques, and how many body systems and conditions that were being activated and helped with proper breathing was very impressive.

Since my practice works with may individuals who have either experienced disease, injury or are living with it, or others whose goal is to improve their health, these techniques can make a different impact and improvement on their health.

Now that I have learned the techniques of the **Optimal Breathing®** Level 1 practitioner, I am very excited to share them with my family, friends and many wonderful clients. — Leiah Carr. March 2002

Counselor in South Africa

I completed my master's degree in counseling. The training course I completed, under the guidance of Michael G White, has added greatly to my counseling resource — just how greatly, the future will tell. In helping my clients to breathe well, I will be opening a door to them to a whole new level of living. How do I know this? From personal experience! As I feel my lungs expanding I believe that I have not only added years to my life, but what I think is even more important, I have added life to my years. — Jerome McCarthy

Preventive Medicine Physician

Breath is the essence of life. When we expire, we lose life. When we are inspired, we gain life. When we form a conspiracy, we plan life together.

The art of optimal breathing can provide a great contribution to the art of optimal living.

Michael Grant White has been studying the science and art of breathing for two decades and is a masterful teacher. His training materials, workshops, and personal coaching sessions provide insights which can transform lives.

I was amazed to learn how much benefit can be gained in chronic diseases such as asthma, angina, emphysema, anxiety, and insomnia thru the application of **Optimal Breathing®** strategies.

I'm glad to be able to endorse Michael Grant White's highly-evolved program of Optimal Breathing. However, as with any program that requires application, the benefits you gain are generally proportional to consistency with which you practice these principles. If you are ready to fulfill your life potential, I recommend you begin by fulfilling your breathing potential. — James Biddle, MD Diplomate, American Board of Internal Medicine; Diplomate, American Board of Chelation Therapy , Asheville NC

Retired Health Care Worker

Optimal Breathing® has changed all my ideas about how to breathe properly and I am glad to be taught by an expert. I wanted to learn how to increase my energy and stamina, and these sessions have also made me aware of what I do to inhibit my breathing and thus limit my energies. H.L. Retired Health Care Worker.

From Candace Pert, author of *Molecules of Emotion*

The peptide-respiratory link is well documented: Virtually any peptide found anywhere else can be found in the respiratory center. This peptide substrate may provide the scientific rationale for the powerful healing effects of consciously controlled breath patterns.

Mind doesn't dominate body; it becomes body. Body and mind are one. I see the process of communication we have demonstrated, the flow of information throughout the whole organism, as evidence that the body is the actual outward manifestation, in physical space of the mind. Bodymind. At this molecular level there really was no distinction between the mind and the body.

From Dr. Erik Peper, author of *Breathing for Health*

Dr. Erik Peper of San Francisco State College has discovered that the most effective way for people to learn to breathe better is through modeling of the action by a skilled therapist or coach.. In the foreword of his book, Chandra Patel, M.D. of the University College London states that *"the two components subjects feel they have benefited from most, and that they are willing to continue using, are awareness of stress and breathing exercises. Human nature makes it unlikely that most people, except those strongly motivated, will comply with a time consuming practice in the long term."*

Chapter 5
RESOURCES

Now you know WHY you need to improve your breathing. I encourage you to take our beginning home study and advanced trainings and become certified to teach others how to improve their breathing. Many health care professionals find breathing development a valuable addition to the services they offer their clients!

You may want to invest in our most popular home study training program *#176 DVD* or *video* (*http://www.breathing.com/video-manual-1-2.htm*) and/or attend the **Optimal Breathing® School** (apprentice and advanced levels) Check our calendar of events for the days and place of the next scheduled **Optimal Breathing® School**: *http://www.breathing.com/school/main.htm*

OUR MOST POPULAR PRODUCTS
Help:
1. **Develop the breathing**
2. **Supportive data to better understand and apply**
3. **Relaxation**
4. **Energizing**
5. **Improve Focus & Concentration.**

1. FIRST develop the breathing to make the fastest largest improvement with the least amount of effort. *#176 DVD/video Fundamentals of Breathing Development:* is GUARANTEED to greatly improve your breathing.
http://www.breathing.com/video-strap.htm

2. Second. Learn about direct and indirect factors aside from rapid breathing development such as stretching, weight training, diet, ergonomics, supportive facts that guide and inspire and much much, more. A distillation of 15 years of full time research of breathing..

#191 Secrets of Optimal Breathing Development –
http://www.breathing.com/secrets.htm

Next: *The Breathing Development 176 program* will often effect an increase in energy and deeper relaxation but is not specifically designed for that. Because of this we recommend that if energy and or relaxation are especially important that you also get either or both:

Exercise #1 **& for Energy** — *Exercise #2.*

    3. Profound Relaxation - #120 *Better Breathing Exercise 1*, *http://www.breathing.com/exercise1.htm*

    4. Balanced Energy - *#130 Better Breathing Exercise 2*, *http://www.breathing.com/exercise2.htm*

    5. Mental focus and concentration – Product #150 .

#150 The Watching Breath guides you in a series of simple but profound ancient mind-body techniques.

There are many others at *http://www.breathing.com/programs.htm,* but we recommend you begin with the ones above.

RECOMMENDED READING
http://www.breathing.com/bibliography.htm

Secrets of Optimal Breathing® Development (includes *Building Healthy Lungs, Naturally*)
http://www.breathing.com/secrets.htm

Breathing for Health by Dr.Erik Peper

Free Your Breath , Free Your Life by Dennis Lewis

http://www.breathing.com/free-your-breath.htm

Flood Your Body with Oxygen by Ed McCabe

Molecules of Emotion by Candace Pert

The Power of Emotion by Michael Sky

The Palette of Breath by Lauren Robins

Unstoppable by Cynthia Kersey

RECOMMENDED WEBSITES

How to CONTACT Mike White

http://www.breathing.com/contact.htm

FREE BREATHING TESTS

http://www.breathing.com/tests.htm

UDB hinders oxygenation & nervous system function

http://www.breathing.com/articles/carbon-dioxide.htm

French study: over 300 Drugs Induce Lung Diseases

http://www.breathing.com/articles/pneumotox.htm

Optimal Breathing® School [a]

http://www.breathing.com/school/main.htm

Find an Optimal Breathing Development Specialist in your area

http://www.breathing.com/school/refer/main.htm

Recommended BOOKS

http://www.breathing.com/bibliography.htm

Recommended breathing PROGRAMS

http://www.breathing.com/programs.htm

Another Optimal Breathing® website

http://www.about-breathing.com

How effective is hyperbaric oxygen therapy

http://www.breathing.com/articles/hyperbaric.htm

Reasonably priced hyperbaric oxygen therapy

http://www.MiracleMountain.org

Fundamentals of breathing development

http://www.breathing.com/video-strap.com

How breathing affects sleep

http://www.breathing.com/sleep-program.htm

New study links sleep deprivation & obesity

http://www.breathing.com/sleep-obesity.htm

"Body Burden" study - how toxins affect health/lungs

http://www.ewg.org

Answers to your questions about local pollution

http://www.scorecard.org

Framingham Study - 50 years of research

http://www.breathing.com/articles/clinical-studies.htm

NADA Chair helps posture for better breathing

http://www.breathing.com/nada.htm

Otto Warburg - Cancer & Oxygen (1930's Nobel Prize winner)

http://www.breathing.com/articles/otto-warburg.htm

Overbreathing: A Major Misconception

http://www.overbreathing.us

"Palette of Breath" by Lauren Robins

http://www.breathing.com/palette.htm

"Flood Your Body with Oxygen" by Ed McCabe

http://www.breathing.com/flood-your-body.htm

Vaccine Dangers

http://www.breathing.com/articles/vaccine-dangers.htm

ALL ABOUT BREATHING. Over 200 articles from A-Z.

http://www.breathing.com/articles/Default.htm

Oxygenized Water

http://www.breathing.com/oxy-water.htm

Leading Cause of Death in the U.S.

http://www.breathing.com/articles/leading-cause-of-death.htm

Announcing the International Breathing Association - now a part of the IMAgroup!

IMA group website

http://www.imagroup.com

Looking for a good MASSAGE, SCHOOLS, SPAS

http://www.ineedamassage.com & http://www.iwantamassage.com

Massage and Oxygen? A wonderful combination!

http://www.oxygenmassage.com

Ozone For Health

http://www.ozoneforhealth.com

Oxygen For Life

http://www.oxygenforlife.org

Oxygen For Health

http://www.oxygenforhealth.com

The Oxygen Center. Soon to be open across the USA

http://www.theoxygencenter.com

All about massage

http://www.aboutmassage.com

Download a FREE PDF of this book! (customize for your bs.!)

http://www.breathing.com/theway.htm

**INEXPENSIVE BLOOD TESTING • HAIR • URINE •
HEAVY METALS NUTRITION & DETOXIFICATION:**
See *Building Healthy Lungs, Naturally*

Information about Building Health Lungs, Naturally

http://www.breathing.com/bhln.htm

How dehydration affects breathing

http://wwwbreathing.com/articles/watercure.htm

In more scientific terms (as defined by Dr. Peter Litchfield
http://www.breathing.com/school/faculty.htm), **how many areas
of <u>your</u> life are affected by the way you breathe?**

*Breath is the beginning and end of life and it has
everything to do with all that's in between.*

**Mike White
The Breathing Coach**® **& OBDS Master Trainer**

Optimal Breathing School
Core Faculty
http://www.breathing.com/school/faculty.htm

Dr. Len Saputo
Donna Gross
Dr. Bill Hoffman
Liz Hoffmaster
Dennis Lewis
Dr. Peter Litchfield

Your improvements on the **Optimal Vitality Goals©** list are best achieved through our Breathing Development Self-Help Programs found at: **http://www.breathing.com/programs.htm** or through personal trainings with an **Optimal Breathing Development Specialist** (find an OBDS in your area at this webpage: **http://www.breathing.com/school/refer.htm**

OPTIMAL BREATHING® SCHOOL

http://www.breathing.com/school.htm

Here's a partial list of modalities that will benefit greatly from attending our school.

Join us and then help us train your colleagues!

Acupressure

Acupuncture

Alexander Technique

Applied Kinesiology

Aromatherapy

Ahashiatsu

Ashtanga Yoga

Aston Patterning

Barbara Brennan Healing Science

Bonnie Prudden Myotherapy

Bowen Bodywork

Brain Gym

Butoh

Canadian Deep Muscle

Chi gung (Qigong)

Chi Nei Tsang

Chiropractors

Colonic Educators

Dance Teachers

Cranio-Sacral

Dance Teachers

Deep Muscle

Energy Field Work

Feldenkrais Method

Feng Shui

Hatha Yoga

Hellerwork

Holotropic breathworkers

Hypnotherapists

Infant massage

Iyengar Yoga

Jin Shin Jyutsu

Jivamukti Yoga

Jois Yoga

Kinesiology

Kripalu Yoga

Kundalini Yoga

Lymph Drainage

Martial arts. Hard and soft styles

Massage therapists & bodyworkers

Medical Doctors

Movement Therapists

Myofascial Release

Neuromuscular

Nurses

Nursing Assistants

Occupational Therapist

Osteopaths

Pain Relief

Personal Trainers

Physical therapists

Psychotherapists

Polarity Therapy

Power Yoga

Prenatal Massage

Psychiatrists

Psychotherapists

Qigong

Radiance breathworkers

Radix

Raja Yoga

Rebirthing

Reichian therapists

Reiki

Reflexology

Respiratory Therapists

Rolfing

Shiatsu

Sivananda Yoga

Speech language pathologists

Stress Relief

Swedish

Tai Ch

Tantra

TCM - Traditional Chinese Medicine

Therapeutic Touch

Three in One

Touch for Health

Transformational breathworkers

Trauma Erase

Trigger Point

Tutoring

Voice and singing teachers

Watsu

Yoga in general

Zero Balancing

http://www.breathing.com/school/main.htm

The Optimal Breathing School.

LEADING EDGE

TOUCH & NON TOUCH METHODS

Learn how + teach others

Rapidly Develop Natural Mechanical Breathing Function

866-694-6425

(866-MyInhale)

mw@breathing.com

http://www.breathing.com/school/main.htm

Accelerating Healthy Breathing & Speech Development

CEUs for Massage Therapists

become an expert in a field few health professionals clearly understand

Mike White's classes address these breathing development problems:

113

- **Weak voice** & unable to project
- **Respiratory illnesses** (i.e. bronchitis, asthma, emphysema
- **Symptomatic problems** (i.e. coughing, chronic fatigue, high blood pressure)
- **Mechanical problems** (i.e. cramps in back or neck, hyperventilation, tightness across chest)
- **Emotional symptoms** (i.e. anxiety, depression, shallow breathing)
- **And everything else** that better breathing can influence or control

You will learn to facilitate significant improvement in your own, as well as most client's, breathing - including asthma, COPD, pulmonary fibrosis, and help improve speaking and singing.

Other benefits can include: improved energy, pain reduction, easing pregnancy and birthing, improved sleep, sports performance, stress management, weight loss, stopping smoking, voice strengthening

Optimal Breathing Maximizes
Health & Well Being
Sports Performance
Life Extension
Helps reduce or eliminate need
for medication!

Health Professionals
Will gain:

Unique Skills • Better Breathing
Grateful Clients • Additional Income
Increased Client Base • Increased Referrals

Our four levels of training
address significant aspects of most
breathing development problems.

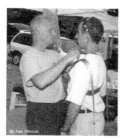 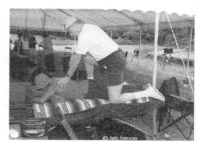

safe * fast * easy * painless

There are many people who have detected breathing problems, such as asthma, COPD, bronchitis — which are easy to spot —but often not easy to improve.

It's the undetected breathing problems that cause the most destruction to a person's health and longevity. These problems act like termites or dry rot because they undermine our vitality and sense of self and allow us to get or stay sick from many other illnesses that use up our oxygen and overtax our nervous, endocrine, digestion, elimination and immune systems.

Take our <u>FREE</u> breathing tests:
http://www.breathing.com/tests.htm

When is the next
Optimal Breathing School[a]
scheduled?

http://www.breathing.com/calendar.htm

Manual & Books

191 - The Secrets of Optimal Breathing
180 page manual. ISBN #188317-48-1 • **$29** + S&H

25 years of research related to poor breathing; anatomy; fundamental & accelerated breathing development; exercises -special situations –175 breathing based holistic health programs, (i.e. asthma, bronchitis, shortness of breath); clinical studies; appendix; testimonials

192 - Building Healthy Lungs, Naturally
Book. ISBN #188317-39-2 • **$15** + S&H

40 page booklet (included in 191 manual or separate) Contains many tips on diet, water, exercise and exercises that can assist you to regain your health and breathing function rapidly. Check out programs:
http://www.breathing.com/programs.htm.

193 - Optimal Breathing®: The Way You Breathe Can Make You Sick! It Can Also Make You Well!
Book. ISBN #188317-06-6 • **$1295** + S&H

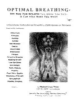

46 page primer that explores conditions or things affecting the quality of your breathing, including: AIR, WATER, FOOD, EXERCISE, EMOTIONS, STRESS TOXINS, TRAUMA. Results from over 40,000 free breathing tests at www.breathing.com show that poor breathing is associated with almost all health challenges! HOW GOOD IS YOUR BREATHING?

DVDs & Videos

176 - **The Art & Science of Optimal Breathing**
DVD or Video - ISBN #188317-41-4 • **$49** pkg + S&H

Developing Healthy Balanced Breathing, About diaphragm, exercises, better sleep & relaxation, pain reduction, reduce medication, ease pregnancy, energy increase, stop smoking, weight loss, sports performance, singing & speaking, tests + Begin HERE.

169 - **Optimal Breathing School**[a]
DVD or video. ISBN #188317-42-2 • **$15** + S&H

For traditional or alternative health professionals, or those aspiring... you MUST learn optimal breathing development. Advanced training levels being added: personal trainers, singers & speakers, specific modality requirements, Qigong masters and more!

194 - **The Way You Breathe Can Make You Sick! It Can Also Make You Well!** DVD or video.
ISBN #188317-47-3 • **$15** + S&H Not available

CDs & Cassettes

120 - **Better Breathing Exercise #1**
CD or cassette. ISBN #188317-44-9 • **$15** + S&H

Deep relaxation and deep letting go; learn to rest more easily and deeply; better access your healing state; become more flexible in your thoughts and actions; handling change in a calmer fashion.

130 - **Better Breathing Exercise #2**
CD or cassette. ISBN #188317-43-0 • **$27** + S&H

Creating natural energy PLUS focus; energetic calm; more life force energy to increase oxygen, nourish brain, enhance cellular function; jump-start metabolism; speed weight loss & recovery from stress & fatigue; boost sexual energy; be more alert yet non-combative.

140 - **Breathing Self Esteem**
CD or cassette. ISBN #188317-46-5 • **$15** + S&H

Increased self understanding, opening to the state of flow, alignment between inner and outer expression, comfort with personal expression; acting on authentic self; less perfectionism.

150 - **The Watching Breath**
180 page manual. ISBN #188317-32-5 • **$15** + S&H

4000-year old meditation - strengthens concentration & deeper awareness; integrating body, breath and mind; better focused thinking; relaxed concentration; calm awareness; opening to a state of slow; being in present time.

170 - **Breath of Life & Vitality**
CD or cassette. ISBN #188317-33-3 • **$15** + S&H

Is there a right way to breathe? Breathing poorly reduces quality of life & life span. Why is deep breathing so misleading to people? Why use inhalers? How to know if you are breathing well? Drug free way to reduce asthma attacks. Importance of nutrition for optimal breathing.

173 - **Raw & Living Foods Festival Seminar**
CD or cassette. ISBN #188317-49-X • **$15** + S&H

Portland, OR- 2001 Festival. Mike delivers a one hour breathing seminar on CD (no cassettes). Fun and very informative. Anatomy, science, why learn to breathe better. Working on a member of the audience.

195 - **The Way You Breathe Can Make You Sick. It Can Also Make You Well!** CD or cassette.

ISBN #188317-10-4 • **$15** + S&H
Not available

Booklets

299 - **Grain Damage**
Booklet   ISBN #1-893831-05-1 • **$7** + S&H

by Dr. Douglas Graham.
Rethinking the high starch diet.
Retail ONLY.

171 - **Optimal Digestion**
Booklet. • **FREE w/orders**

40 page booklet (included in 191 manual or separate) Contains many programs. http://www.breathing.com/programs.htm.

E3Live Super Booster Food
Booklet. • **FREE w/orders**

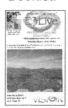

FREE information and bonus gift with first order!
http://www.breathing.com/e3live.htm

Forty-nine Tips
Booklet. • **$5** + S&H (or included with 250 orders)

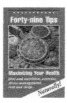

49 great tips on diet and nutrition, exercise, stress management and rest. Start living the healthful life of your dreams today!   From the editors of *Health Science* ® magazine - health & dietary principles available nowhere else.

More CDs & Cassettes

181 - **Prevention & Intention**
CD or cassette. ISBN #188317-28-7 • **$15** + S&H

> Deep relaxation and deep letting go; learn to rest more easily and deeply; better access your healing state; become more flexible in your thoughts and actions; handling change in a calmer fashion.

130 - **Rip Roaring Health**
CD or cassette. ISBN #188317-36-8 • **$15** + S&H

> Creating natural energy PLUS focus; energetic calm; more life force energy to increase oxygen, nourish brain, enhance cellular function; jump-start metabolism; speed weight loss & recovery from stress & fatigue; boost sexual energy; be more alert yet non-combative.

160 - **Peace Within**
CD or cassette. ISBN #188317-30-9 • **$15** + S&H

> Opening to the state of flow; peace of mind; sense of well being; improved creativity; decrease anxiety, tension and aggressiveness.

179 - **Better, deeper, more restful sleep**
CD or cassette. ISBN #188317-09-0 • **$15** + S&H

> Techniques, exercises, ergonomics, nutrition. Comes with 8-page sheet of facts about sleep.

Use our comprehensive way of evaluating your breathing:
FREE BREATHING TESTS: http://*www.breathing.com/tests.htm*

Wholesale orders — 10 minimum of any
60% cost of retail price
plus 7% for quantity shipping in USA.
Call about international shipping rates.
CREDIT CARDS Accepted:
VISA • MasterCard » American Express • Discover

http://www.breathing.com/programs.htm
USA Toll Free: 1-866-694-6425
International 828-456-5689
Fax 828-454-5475
P.O. Box 1551 • Waynesville, NC 28786

Unit Prices
#176 DVD & Video - $49 (package)
#169 OB School - DVD or Video- $15
CDs - $15 • Cassettes - $12
Manual - $29

Qty	Product	Unit $	Total $
____	191 Secrets Manual	$29	_____
____	190 TWYB Book	$1295	_____
____	192 BHLN Book	$15	_____
____	176 Art OB DVD ____ Video ____	$49 pkg	_____
____	169 OB Sch DVD ____ Video ___	$15/12	_____
____	194 TWYB DVD ___	$15	_____
____	120 BBE#1 CD __ Cass __	$15	_____
____	130 BBE#2 CD __ Cass __	$27	_____
____	140 Self Est. CD__ Cass__	$15	_____
____	150 Watch Br. CD __ Cass __	$15	_____
____	170 Br. of Life CD __ Cass __	$15	_____
____	173 Raw Seminar CD __ Cass 195	$15	_____
____	OB CD __ Cass __	$15	_____
	CIRCLE ITEMS THIS PAGE		

This Primer Exposes:

- **Breathing Problems Begin BEFORE Pregnancy**
- **Conditions or things that affect the quality of your breathing include:**
AIR • WATER • FOOD • EXERCISE • EMOTIONS • STRESS • TOXINS • TRAUMA
- **Myths & Cautions About Breathing**
- **What to do if you already have breathing problems**

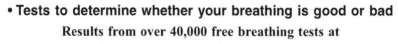

- **Tests to determine whether your breathing is good or bad**

Results from over 40,000 free breathing tests at

http://www.breathing.com/tests.htm

show that poor breathing is associated with almost <u>all</u> health challenges!

HOW GOOD IS YOUR BREATHING?

Breath is the essence of life. When we expire, we lose life. When we are inspired, we gain life. When we form a community, we plan life and breathe together. The art of Optimal Breathing® can provide a great contribution to the art of optimal living. — **Dr. James Biddle, Asheville, NC**

I was amazed to learn how much benefit can be gained in chronic diseases such as asthma, angina, emphysema, anxiety, and insomnia thru the application of Optimal Breathing® strategies. — **J.K., NYC**

I've been searching for better breathing information for a long-time, taking yoga classes for many years, reading books on pranayama & breathing workshops. ...your program is the best I've ever seen! I was feeling exhausted this morning and no amount of rest helped. I did some of your breathing exercises and felt energized. — **Dave K., Chicago**

GUARANTEED IMPROVEMENT Techniques introduced in this book integrate the natural breathing reflex of ALL key areas of mechanical breathing function: diaphragm, abdominal, lower, mid & upper back, right & left sides & upper chest - with the appropriate accessory breathing muscles. This increases vital capacity PLUS increases voice strength and sound.